Key Concepts in Traditional Chinese Medicine II

Li Zhaoguo • Wu Qing • Xing Yurui

Key Concepts in Traditional Chinese Medicine II

palgrave
macmillan

Li Zhaoguo
Shanghai Normal University
Shanghai, China

Wu Qing
Beijing University of Chinese Medicine
Beijing, China

Xing Yurui
Shaanxi University of Chinese
Medicine
Shaan Xi, China

ISBN 978-981-16-2397-4   ISBN 978-981-16-2398-1   (eBook)
https://doi.org/10.1007/978-981-16-2398-1

Jointly published with Foreign Language Teaching and Research Publishing Co., Ltd
The print edition is not for sale in China (Mainland). Customers from China (Mainland)
please order the print book from: Foreign Language Teaching and Research Publishing
Co., Ltd.

This Palgrave Macmillan imprint is published by the registered company Springer Nature
Singapore Pte Ltd.
The registered company address is: 152 Beach Road, #21-01/04 Gateway East, Singapore
189721, Singapore

PREFACE

TCM, short for traditional Chinese medicine, is a classical medical system with Chinese characteristics that are closely integrated with astronomy, geography, and humanities. Based on traditional Chinese culture, classical philosophy, and humanistic thoughts, TCM, in combination with the various schools of thought and their exponents during the period from pre-Qin times to the early years of the Han Dynasty as well as the theories and practice of natural sciences and social sciences, constitutes the unique theoretical system, way of thinking, and diagnosis and treatment methods. TCM has a high regard for the harmonious coexistence of man and nature. It emphasizes consistent cultural inheritance, advocates the harmonious development between man and society, and opens broad prospects for local medicine development, cultural dissemination, and the progress of human civilization. As promulgated in the white paper "Traditional Chinese Medicine in China" by the State Council in 2016, TCM is a "representative feature of Chinese civilization," which "produces a positive impact on the progress of human civilization," "represents a combination of natural sciences and humanities," and "embraces profound philosophical ideas of the Chinese nation."

TCM is a comprehensive and widely used traditional medical system in the world with a long history. It is characterized by profound culture, distinctive effects, and fast development. Early in the pre-Qin period, TCM had been gradually introduced into the neighboring areas such as the Korean Peninsula. During the Han and Tang dynasties, it had been brought into Japan and Southeast Asia. After the eighteenth century,

TCM was introduced into Europe and it gained wide dissemination in the mid-nineteenth century. After the 1970s, TCM quickly spread all over the world along with the success of acupuncture anesthesia, contributing substantially to the development of world medicine, the well-being of all nations, and the dissemination of Chinese culture. Due to its advanced theory, profound cultural basis, natural therapy, and remarkable effectiveness, TCM has survived and prospered throughout the ages. It has blazed a unique path for the prosperity of the Chinese nation, the development of Chinese civilization, and the spread of Chinese culture.

Four TCM classics—*Yellow Emperor's Internal Canon of Medicine, Canon of Difficult Issues, Agriculture God's Canon of Materia Medica*, and *Treatise on Cold Damage and Miscellaneous Diseases*—not only represent the core of TCM theory and method but also contain the essence of thought and spirit in Chinese culture, among which *Yellow Emperor's Internal Canon of Medicine* is the landmark. It involves almost every aspect of natural sciences, social sciences, and language and culture in ancient China. Its worldwide spread has become a great way for Chinese culture to go global. The transliteration form of the important concepts of Chinese culture such as yin, yang, and qi has been adopted in Western languages. This is a great contribution made by TCM to the "going out" of Chinese culture, and it has laid a solid language foundation for Chinese culture going out.

Chinese culture is going to spread to the West, to the world. Naturally, there is a need for attention from various academic, cultural, and civil sectors. In the Han and Tang dynasties, the Buddhists in Xiyu (the Western regions) traveled all the way to Central China to promote Buddhism, whereas in the Ming and Qing dynasties Western missionaries worked their way to China to spread Christianity. For both of them, medicine has been an important means to rally public support. As an integral part of traditional Chinese culture, TCM not only plays an important role in rallying foreign support to stimulate Chinese culture to go global but also serves as a bridge to disseminate and promote traditional Chinese culture directly. It is an international consensus that anyone desiring to learn, understand, and draw on TCM theories, methods, formulas, and herbs shall first of all learn and acquire the basic theories and thoughts of traditional Chinese culture, for example, the theory of yin and yang, the theory of five elements, and the theory of essence and qi.

It can be seen that the international communication of TCM is undoubtedly an ideal, unique, and solid approach if Chinese culture is to go global in a comprehensive and systematic manner and to gain the heartfelt understanding and acceptance from the people worldwide.

Shanghai, China   Li Zhaoguo
Beijing, China   Wu Qing
Shaan Xi, China   Xing Yurui

NOTE TO READERS

The *Key Concepts in Traditional Chinese Medicine* published in May 2018 includes 111 very basic terms concerning the thoughts and culture of traditional Chinese medicine (TCM), mainly related to essence, qi, the theory of yin and yang, five elements, and visceral manifestation. This book covers 110 terms related to visceral manifestation, meridians, etiology, pathogenesis, and treatment principles, providing simplified Chinese characters, Mandarin pronunciation in pinyin, English translation of the term, definitions, previous translation of the term (used before year 2000), current translation of the term (used after year 2000), standard translation of the term, and citations from TCM classics. A list of concepts, index, and reference books are placed at the very end of this book. It is expected that readers not only understand the Chinese meaning and English translation of the terms but also gain a deeper understanding of the progress made over a period of 40 years in the studies of TCM term translation by comparing their "previous translation" with their "current translation." In addition, readers can gain an insight into the specific application of the included terms by referring to their corresponding citations. This book can be a helpful resource to the readers at home and abroad who want to learn, understand, and draw on the fundamental concepts in TCM. It may serve as valuable reference material for the readers who would like to engage in the English translation of TCM texts, the international communication of Chinese culture, and the research of TCM literature.

Contents

Key Concepts in Traditional Chinese Medicine II

Abstract The *Key Concepts in Traditional Chinese Medicine* published in May 2018 includes 111 very basic terms concerning the thoughts and culture of traditional Chinese medicine (TCM), mainly related to essence, qi, the theory of yin and yang, five elements, and visceral manifestation. This book covers 110 key concepts related to visceral manifestation, meridians, etiology, pathogenesis, therapeutic principles and methods in traditional Chinese medicine, providing simplified Chinese characters, Mandarin pronunciation in pinyin, definitions, and citations. A variety of English versions of each term or concept over a period of 40 years is offered before a standard English version is proposed upon an examination of the connotation of the Chinese term and English vocabulary, making it possible for the readers to become aware of the translation history of traditional Chinese medicine. Readers who are familiar with or keen on learning traditional Chinese medicine to communicate across cultures can have a source for either speaking or writing these terms. This book can be a helpful resource to understand the fundamental terms of traditional Chinese medicine and culture.

Keywords Traditional Chinese medicine • Thoughts and culture • Term translation

1. TIĀN RÉN HÉYĪ 天人合一

Oneness of Heaven and Human

The term refers to a concept in traditional Chinese thought, that is, the unity of heaven and human, of the way of heaven and the way of human, and of nature and human. It is an important proposition of ancient Chinese philosophy with its varied meanings in different historical contexts. From the perspective of traditional Chinese medicine (TCM), it mainly denotes that man and nature are homologous, that is, all things in the universe including human beings are derived from original qi. In addition, man and nature are isomorphic, that is, all things in the universe including human beings are of the same structure composed of original qi, yin, yang, the five elements, and so on. Finally, man and nature follow identical laws, that is, man and nature observe similar principles of waxing and waning of yin and yang as well as the principles of generation, restriction, inhibition, and transformation among the five elements.

As the core of traditional Chinese culture, the concept of heaven-human oneness defines the universe as the realm of human existence; thus, it stipulates the physical attributes, the value orientation, the realm of life, and the dimension of transcendence as well as the way of understanding and thinking of human beings. This concept is then borrowed and further developed as the epistemology, methodology, and value system for the construction of theoretical system and the guidance of clinical practice of TCM.

[**Previous Translation**] Unite the nature with human being; human body corresponds to the nature
[**Current Translation**] Unity of the heaven and humanity; holistic view of the heaven and environment
[**Standard Translation**] Oneness of heaven and human

Citations

- Man follows the laws of nature, and corresponds to the working principles of the sun and the moon. (*Spiritual Pivot*)
- Man depends on the heaven qi and the earth qi for existence and lives in accordance with the principle of the four seasons. (*Plain Conversation*)
- Confucianists, on the other hand, have a clear understanding of the heavenly principle by observing human relations, and thus under-

stand worldly affairs by referring to the heavenly principle. Therefore, man and heaven are united in oneness. Man can become sages through learning, having both a command of the heavenly principle and an insight into human relations. (*Enlightenment Through Confucian Teachings*)

2. XÍNG SHÉN YĪTǏ 形神一体

Unity of Body and Spirit

The term refers to an important proposition of ancient Chinese philosophy and traditional Chinese medicine (TCM) concerning the relationship between physiology and psychology. "Body" refers to the physical aspect, that is, zang-fu organs and physical form; "spirit" refers to the spiritual aspect, that is, mental activities characterized by the five spirits and the five emotions. In TCM, body and spirit are an inseparable unity. They go hand in hand to flourish alike or to perish together. Spirit is born from and dependent on physical body for existence. Residing in physical body, spirit will be vigorous when one is physically abundant and exhaustive when one is physically diminished. Their relationship was summarized in the "Discussion on Ancient Innocence Theory" of *Plain Conversation* as the "harmony between body and spirit," which marked the establishment of the materialist concept of body and spirit. While affirming the physical body determines spirit, it also emphasizes the dominance of spirit over body. It is believed that the coordination of the functions of the zang-fu organs and their adaptation to the external natural and social environments are inseparable from the regulation of spirit.

[**Previous Translation**] Unity of body and spirit
[**Current Translation**] Unity of physique and spirit; unity of body and spirit; integration of body and spirit
[**Standard Translation**] Unity of body and spirit

Citations

- That is why they could maintain harmony and unity of body and spirit, enjoying good health and long life. (*Plain Conversation*)
- Form is the vehicle for spirit, and spirit is the embodiment of form. Without spirit, form is lifeless; without form, spirit shall not come into being. (*Classified Classics*)

3. Jūnzhǔ zhī guān 君主之官

Monarch

The term refers to a ruler running an empire. In traditional Chinese medicine, the heart governs the mental activity as well as the physiological activities of all organs and tissues in humans. For one thing, the heart governs the mind and regulates various mental activities. As stated in the "Diseases" section of *Classified Classics*, "the heart, being the monarch of the five zang-organs and six fu-organs, commands ethereal soul and corporeal soul, and involves will." For another, it is vital for the heart to coordinate different physiological functions of all organs for the fulfillment of overall life activities. The heart performs the function of governing all human life activities, hence the metaphorical term used in the "Discussion on the Secret Canons Stored in Royal Library" of *Plain Conversation*.

[**Previous Translation**] Office of monarch; Heart; monarch organ; organ as monarch
[**Current Translation**] Monarch organ; monarch-organ; king-organ; key organ; heart, which is the organ similar to the monarch
[**Standard Translation**] Monarch

Citations

- The heart governs the life activities of the whole body, so its role is likened to that of a monarch. (*Essentials of the Internal Canon of Medicine*)
- The monarch is the ruler of a state. As far as the twelve zang-fu organs are concerned, the heart is regarded as the monarch. (*Direct Interpretation of Plain Conversation in Yellow Emperor's Internal Canon of Medicine*)

4. XIÀNGFÙ ZHĪ GUĀN 相傅之官

Prime Minister

The term refers to the official position of a prime minister or honored ministers such as *taifu* (太傅, literally grandmaster) and *shaofu* (少傅, literally junior master) who assist the monarch in governing the empire. According to traditional Chinese medicine, the lung governs qi and its dispersion, depuration, and descent. Besides, the lung is where all meridians and vessels converge. With these functions, it assists the heart in regulating the functional activities of the whole body in the same manner that the prime minister assists the monarch in governing the empire. Hence the role of the lung is likened to that of the prime minister according to the section "Discussion on the Secret Canons Stored in Royal Library" of *Plain Conversation*. Specifically, the lung is involved in the following functions. First, the lung governs rhythmical respiration, controls the rhythm of breathing, and therefore regulates the generation of pectoral qi, nutrient qi, and defense qi. Second, through dispersion, depuration, and descent, the lung regulates the ascending, descending, exiting, and entering of qi, including the qi in zang-fu organs and meridians, pectoral qi, nutrient qi, and defense qi. Third, the lung governs qi, through which it promotes and regulates blood circulation, and helps to maintain normal heart rhythm and heart rate. Fourth, the lung governs dispersion, depuration, and descent of qi, through which it regulates the distribution and excretion of body fluids.

[**Previous Translation**] Lung
[**Current Translation**] Official acting as the prime minister
[**Standard Translation**] Prime minister

Citations

- Both the lung and the heart are in the chest and above the diaphragm. The lung is positioned high, close to the heart—the monarch. It is likened to the prime minister, hence the metaphorical name. (*Classified Classics*)
- The lung is positioned high in the human body like a "florid canopy." It is likened to the prime minister, housing ethereal soul and governing the qi in the whole body. (*Commentary on the "Agriculture God's Canon of Materia Medica"*)

5. JIĀNGJŪN ZHĪ GUĀN 将军之官

General

The term refers to a high rank of officer in the army. As described in the "Discussion on the Secret Canons Stored in Royal Library" of *Plain Conversation*, it is a metaphor, indicating the role of the liver is likened to that of a senior military commander-in-chief, devising strategies with bravery and wisdom. The liver is the unyielding zang-organ, which prefers free activity and detests depression. Its qi easily becomes hyperactive, like the general being righteous and bold. The liver governs the coursing of qi, regulates emotions, and is involved in mental activities. It corresponds to *shaoyang* upward-rising spring qi, thus full of vitality. Consequently, the liver governs such mental activities as planning and strategizing. If the liver fails to govern planning, such symptoms will occur as poor sense of strategy, retardation, being slow in words and deeds, foolhardiness, vexation, irritability, or even madness.

[**Previous Translation**] Liver; general organ; organ as general
[**Current Translation**] General-like organ (liver)
[**Standard Translation**] General

Citations

- It is brave and decisive, hence the name "general." (*Plain Conversation in Yellow Emperor's Internal Canon of Medicine Annotated by Wang Bing*)
- The liver governs anger. It is so named as general officer by analogy. When people are angry, they lose the ability to plan well, which is a manifestation of the liver disorder. Therefore, in consideration of the symptoms that occur from dysfunction, the liver is believed to govern strategy-making when it functions properly. (*Record of Wisdom Observed in the Medical Classics*)

6. CĀNGLǏN ZHĪ GUĀN 倉廩之官

Granary Officer

The term refers to the official in charge of the granary. It is a metaphor for the functions of the spleen and the stomach in taking in and transporting food and drinks as well as transforming them into essence. Specifically, the stomach receives, stores, and decomposes food, while the spleen governs transportation and transformation. Their functions are closely associated with each other. They cooperate: the ingested food and drinks are decomposed by the stomach, then transported and transformed by the spleen into essential qi, blood, and body fluids before being further transmitted to the whole body to nourish the five zang-organs, six fu-organs, limbs, and bones. The spleen and the stomach work in the same way a granary provides man with food, hence comes the metaphorical name in the "Discussion on the Secret Canons Stored in Royal Library" of *Plain Conversation*. If the functions of the spleen and the stomach are vigorous, sources of nutrients will be abundant; otherwise, the generation of essential qi, blood, and body fluids will be insufficient, and symptoms such as lassitude, fatigue, shortness of breath, no desire to speak, dizziness, as well as emaciation can occur.

[**Previous Translation**] Office of the granary (referring to the spleen and stomach); SPLEEN AND STOMACH ARE THE WARE-HOUSE; official of the granaries; barn official; barn organ; spleen and stomach
[**Current Translation**] Barn organ; barn official (spleen and stomach); organ of granary
[**Standard Translation**] Granary officer

Citations

- The spleen governs the transportation and transformation of food and drinks, and the stomach receives them. Both are in charge, so the spleen and the stomach are described as granary officers. (*Classified Classics*)
- The spleen ... is the root of the granary which stores food and drinks and is the place where nutrient qi is generated... Spleen manifests its condition in the luster of lips, and it helps to strengthen muscles. (*Plain Conversation*)

7. ZUÒQIÁNG ZHĪ GUĀN 作强之官

Labor Officer

The term refers to the official in charge of work requiring laborious efforts (such as building and handicraft making). The kidney stores essence as well as governs growth, development, and reproduction. The essence generates marrow whose functions are two-fold. On the one hand, the marrow nourishes bones. If the kidney essence is abundant, one has strong bones and physical strength, with light but forceful movements. On the other hand, the marrow helps nourish brain—the sea of marrows. If kidney essence is abundant, the sea of marrow will be full and the original spirit will be nourished, then one will be smart, witty, and skillful. Therefore, the kidney is described as a "labor officer and it is responsible for skills" in the "Discussion on the Secret Canons Stored in Royal Library" of *Plain Conversation*. If little attention is paid to health preservation, for example, sexual overindulgence, kidney-essence depletion might occur, in which case the bones and marrow will be deprived of nourishment, causing such symptoms as soreness and weakness of waist and knees, weak limbs, fatigue, dizziness, tinnitus, and even memory loss.

[**Previous Translation**] Office of labor; kidney
[**Current Translation**] The organ in charge of agility; kidney
[**Standard Translation**] Labor officer

Citations

- The kidney pertains to water. It stores essence which forms the foundation of the human body. When essence becomes abundant and the body matures, body function and physical health are well kept, hence the metaphorical name labor officer. (*Classified Classics*)
- The kidney pertains to water according to the five-element theory and corresponds to north. It governs bones, thus named as "labor officer." Water is believed to transform and generate all things, hence the saying "the kidney is responsible for skills." (*Essentials of the Internal Canon of Medicine*)

8. ZHŌNGZHÈNG ZHĪ GUĀN 中正之官

Justice Officer

Zhongzheng (中正, literally middle and rightness) means fairness and impartiality. The gallbladder is situated in the middle of the zang-fu organs, and its meridian is located in the half exterior and the half interior, like the "middle" position of the second or the fifth line in a *Yi* hexagram, hence called *zhong* (中, middle). In addition, the gallbladder stores bile and is involved in the mental activities. It is both an extraordinary organ and one of the six fu-organs characterized by discharge without storage. The gallbladder has the attributes of both yin and yang, with dual functions of storage and discharge, like the yang lines in the yang position (the first, third, or fifth line) or the yin lines in the yin position (the second, fourth, or sixth line) in a *Yi* hexagram, hence called *zheng* (正, rightness or exactness). The liver and the gallbladder are closely connected in functions: the former governs strategy-making; the latter controls decision-making in order to make a sound judgment, hence comes the name "justice officer" in the "Discussion on the Secret Canons Stored in Royal Library" of *Plain Conversation*. If the gallbladder qi is weak, gallbladder dysfunction occurs in terms of decision-making. As a result, mental and emotional disorders such as timidity, fright, fear, insomnia, and dreaminess may occur.

[**Previous Translation**] Official acting as a mediator; office of justice; gallbladder
[**Current Translation**] The official acting as a mediator; gallbladder; fu-viscera with decisive character
[**Standard Translation**] Justice officer

Citations

- It is upright and resolute, honest and assertive, hence the metaphorical name justice officer. (*Plain Conversation in Yellow Emperor's Internal Canon of Medicine Annotated by Wu Kun*)
- According to the "Discussion on Six-plus-six System and the Manifestations of the Viscera" in *Plain Conversation*, all functions of eleven zang-fu organs depend on the normal function of the gallbladder, which means each of the zang-fu organs has its respective

functions, and the gallbladder regulates them, judging right from wrong, making impartial decisions, hence the saying "the gallbladder is the justice officer." (*Adapted Interpretation of Plain Conversation in Yellow Emperor's Internal Canon of Medicine*)

9. ZHŌUDŪ ZHĪ GUĀN 州都之官

Reservoir Officer

Originally *zhoudu* (州都, literally state and capital) refers to a habitable place in the water. Here it is a metaphor for the role of the urinary bladder in governing the storage and discharge of water. The body fluids as a result of metabolism are transmitted to the urinary bladder. With kidney's function of qi transformation, the lucidity ascends and the turbidity descends. The lucid is vaporized and then transmitted to the whole body through triple energizer; the turbid is transformed into urine and then discharged from the urethra. According to the section "Discussion on Zang-fu Pathogenesis" of *Treatise on Blood Syndromes* written by Tang Rongchuan in the Qing Dynasty (1616–1911), "*The Internal Canon of Medicine* says that as a result of the qi transformation of the urinary bladder, water is discharged and carried upward and outward, which is manifested as sweat...." This indicates that the discharge of water including sweat and urine is related to the qi-transformation function of the urinary bladder, hence the quotation "the urinary bladder is the reservoir officer and is responsible for storing and discharging water by means of qi transformation" in the "Discussion on the Secret Canons Stored in Royal Library" of *Plain Conversation.*

[**Previous Translation**] THE OFFICIAL MANAGING THE RESERVOIR; river island official; Regional Rectifier; bladder
[**Current Translation**] Bladder
[**Standard Translation**] Reservoir officer

Citations

- The urinary bladder governs water and is the place where the fluids are stored, hence the name reservoir officer. (*Collective Annotations of Plain Conversation in Yellow Emperor's Internal Canon of Medicine*)

- The urinary bladder is at the bottom of the abdominal cavity where the water in triple energizer gathers, like a reservoir. Hence it is named reservoir officer, responsible for storing fluids. (*Classified Classics*)

10. CHUÁNDÀO ZHĪ GUĀN 传道之官

Transportation Officer

The large intestine is likened to an official in charge of transporting goods. It, including the sigmoid colon and the rectum, joins the small intestine at the ileocolic opening and ends at the anus. Receiving the undigested substances from the small intestine, the large intestine is primarily involved in the absorption of water and nutrients from food residues, forming feces, and defecation. It is this important function of transporting the waste substances that gives it the name transportation officer, which was written in the "Discussion on the Secret Canons Stored in Royal Library" of *Plain Conversation*. Disorders such as constipation or diarrhea are commonly reported if the large intestine fails to perform its transportation task.

[**Previous Translation**] Official in charge of transportation (large intestine); official in charge of transportation; transportation official; office of conveyance; organ with the function of transmission
[**Current Translation**] The organ in charge of transportation; organ in charge of transmission; transportation organ (large intestine); organ responsible for conveyance; official of transportation; officer in charge of transportation
[**Standard Translation**] Transportation officer

Citations

- The large intestine starts from the terminal point of the small intestine. Its primary function includes the removal of waste substances, which involves conversion and transportation. (*Essentials of the Internal Canon of Medicine*)
- The reason why the large intestine can transport waste substances is that it is closely related to the lung. The lung governs descent of qi,

so the large intestine can transport wastes. Hence it is necessary to regulate lung qi for the regulation of defecation. (*Essentials of Integrated Traditional Chinese and Western Medicine*)

11. JUÉDÚ ZHĪ GUĀN 决渎之官

Drainage Officer

The term refers to the official responsible for dredging waterways, meaning the job of triple energizer is to dredge water passage and transport water. The distribution and excretion of human body fluids is completed through the synergistic function of different organs including the lung, the spleen, and the kidney, which is only made possible when triple energizer serves as the water passage and its qi serves as the driving force. If triple energizer fails to perform its function, it becomes difficult for the lung, the spleen, and the kidney to regulate water metabolism, which may result in less urine, edema, and other pathological changes. According to the "Discussion on the Secret Canons Stored in Royal Library" of *Plain Conversation*, "triple energizer is the drainage officer and is responsible for regulating the pathway for water transport in the whole body."

[**Previous Translation**] The official who manages the dredging of water (triple warmer); the official managing the dredging of water pathway; the irrigation official who builds waterways; water-course dredging official; organ for water excretion

[**Current Translation**] The organ in charge of water circulation; organ in charge of water drainage (triple energizer); organ for water excretion; triple energizer

[**Standard Translation**] Drainage officer

Citations

- The function of the upper energizer is like fog, the middle energizer a fermentor, and the lower energizer a drainer. Therefore, triple energizer is like a drainage officer, bringing the water in the upper and middle energizers to the lower energizer, thus forming the passage for water discharge. (*Direct Interpretation of Plain Conversation in Yellow Emperor's Internal Canon of Medicine*)

- *Jue* (决) means dredging and *du* (渎) means waterways. Water will attack the heart and the lung if the upper energizer fails to perform its functions; water retention will occur in the spleen and stomach if the middle energizer fails to play its role; urine and defecation disorders will arise if the lower energizer does not work properly. When the qi in triple energizer keeps harmony, the meridians will be unblocked and the flow of waterways will be smooth, hence the name "drainage officer" for triple energizer. (*Classified Classics*)

12. YUÁNSHÉN ZHĪ FǓ 元神之府

House of Original Spirit

The term refers to the place for accommodating original spirit. Original spirit, also known as inborn spirit, is what develops from the embryo as a result of sperm-egg binding. The brain is primarily involved in governing life activities, mental activities, senses, and movements. It stores original spirit and provides material basis for its activities. Hence the brain is called the "house of original spirit." According to the "Discussion on the Spirit of Human Body" of *Records of Chinese Medicine with Reference to Western Medicine* written by Zhang Xichun, "The brain houses original spirit; the heart governs conscious spirit that is acquired later. Original spirit in the brain is natural, void, and bright, free from meditation and deliberation, whereas conscious spirit in the heart involves meditation and deliberation, and is bright but not void." Higher levels of mental activities such as thinking, consciousness, and emotions are based on both original spirit and conscious spirit and are jointly regulated by the brain and the heart through analyzing, planning, and memorizing objective things in the world. Therefore, original spirit is extremely important for life activities. Life exists with original spirit and ends without it.

[**Previous Translation**] Supreme mental palace (brain); THE RESIDENCE OF MIND; the palace of the mind; the house of primordial mind; house of the original spirit; house of mental activity; brain

[**Current Translation**] House of mental activities; house of cerebral spirit; brain; house of mentality; seat of mental activity; fu-viscera of mental activity; house of (the) original spirit

[**Standard Translation**] House of original spirit

Citations

- The brain is where original spirit is housed, whereas the nose is the orifice of life gate. (*Compendium of Materia Medica*)
- The brain is where original spirit stays and where essence converges. In fact, memory relies on the brain. (*Categorized Patterns with Clear-Cut Treatments*)
- The brain is where original spirit stays and where lucid yang converges. (*Medical Law Tact*)

13. SHĒNGJIÀNG CHŪRÙ 升降出入

Ascending, Descending, Exiting, and Entering

The term refers to the four basic forms of qi movement. Ascending and descending are the upward and downward movements of qi, while exiting and entering are the outward and inward movements of qi. There is a variety of forms of qi movement, including the pair of opposites such as ascending and descending, exiting and entering, attracting and repelling, spreading and condensing. Traditional Chinese medicine focuses on the qi movement of ascending, descending, exiting, and entering, believing that "nothing can exist without qi movement." Ascending and descending as well as exiting and entering of qi are contradictory movements of the unity of opposites, which are extensively present in the human body. For one thing, ascending versus descending and exiting versus entering, as well as ascending and descending versus exiting and entering, are mutually restrictive and mutually reinforcing, thus maintaining harmony. For another, although a certain form of qi movement has dominance over a certain organ, for example, the liver and the spleen are primarily involved in ascending qi, while the lung and the stomach are primarily involved in descending qi, the balance between ascending and descending, exiting and entering must be coordinated from a holistic perspective of the human body. Only in this way can qi movement and visceral functions in the human body be normal. Therefore, a coordinated balance of qi movement, that is, ascending and descending, exiting and entering, plays an important part in maintaining normal life activities.

[**Previous Translation**] Ascending, descending, exiting, entering; ascending-descending and coming in-going out

[**Current Translation**] Ascending, descending, out-going, and in-going; ascending, descending, exiting, and entering; ascending, descending, going out, and coming in; upward, downward, inward, and outward movement

[**Standard Translation**] Ascending, descending, exiting, and entering

Citations

- When qi ceases exiting and entering, vital activities shall vanish; when qi ceases ascending and descending, qi configuration shall perish. Therefore, without exiting-entering of qi, there will be no birth, growth, maturity, senility, or death; without ascending-descending of qi, there will be no germination, growth, flowering, reaping, or storage. Consequently, ascending, descending, exiting, and entering of qi are found in every form of life. (*Plain Conversation*)
- There is no exiting-entering of qi if there is no ascending-descending of qi, and vice versa. Ascending-descending and exiting-entering are important to each other. (*Random Notes While Reading About Medicine*)

14. JĪNXUÈ TÓNGYUÁN 津血同源

Body Fluids and Blood Are of the Same Origin

The term means that both body fluids and blood are derived from the essence of food and drinks. They are of the same source. They nourish, transform, and affect each other. First, both body fluids and blood are liquids, pertaining to yin. They originate from the essence of food and drinks and are transported and transformed by the stomach and the spleen. They moisten and nourish each other, and jointly nourish the human body. Second, body fluids and blood can transform into each other in the course of circulation and distribution. Body fluids are transformed into blood when they enter the blood vessels; water in the blood seeps out of the vessels and is transformed into body fluids. It is precisely because of the close relationship between body fluids and blood that they affect each other in terms of pathogenesis. For example, excessive blood loss may damage body fluids, resulting in thirst, less urine, dry skin, and other pathological changes. Conversely, serious damage of body fluids will also affect the blood, causing blood deficiency, exhaustion of body fluids, blood dryness, and so on.

[**Previous Translation**] Body fluid and blood are derived from the same source; The body fluid and blood are of the same origin; Body fluid and the blood are derived from the same source; Liquid and blood are of the same source

[**Current Translation**] Body fluid and blood derived from the same source; Body fluids and blood are derived from a common source; body fluid and blood sharing the same origin/source; body fluids and blood being of the same source; homogeny of clear fluid and blood; homogeny of fluid and blood; fluid and blood from same source

[**Standard Translation**] Body fluids and blood are of the same origin.

Citations

- The nutrient-qi is transformed in the middle energizer. Like fog and dew, it enters the interstitial space, infuses into the minute collaterals, and blends in the body fluids before being transformed into blood. (*Spiritual Pivot*)
- Body fluids are the surplus of blood, which flow outside the blood vessels and circulate throughout the human body like clean dew in nature. (*Miscellaneous Writings of Famous Physicians of the Ming Dynasty*)
- Food and drinks can be transformed into body fluids, in which the thick part is blood and the thin part is fluid. The fluids are what moisten the zang-fu organs, muscles, and blood vessels so that qi and blood can flow smoothly without impediment. (*Random Notes While Reading About Medicine*)

15. xuèhàn tóngyuán 血汗同源

Blood and Sweat Are of the Same Origin

The term means that both blood and sweat originate from food and drinks and are dependent on the transformation of body fluids. According to traditional Chinese medicine, blood is composed of nutrient-qi and body fluids, in which the part that seeps out of the blood vessels is transformed into body fluids. Body fluids are turned into sweat when they evaporate to skin under the steaming function of yang-qi, hence the saying "blood and sweat are of the same origin." The saying suggests that excessive sweat damages not only body fluids but also blood; and the loss of blood damages not only body fluids but also sweat. Therefore, for hemorrhagic patients, sweating method should be avoided; otherwise, body fluids will be seriously damaged and the condition worsens. In cases of excessive sweating and fluid deficiency, bloodletting and removing blood stasis by drastic methods should be avoided; otherwise, body fluids and blood will be seriously damaged and the condition will worsen. Therefore, according to Zhang Zhongjing's *Treatise on Cold Damage*, "sweating therapy should be avoided in patients with nosebleeds" and "sweating therapy should be avoided in cases of blood exhaustion."

[**Previous Translation**] Blood and sweat are derived from the same source; Blood and sweat share the same source; Blood and sweat have the same source

[**Current Translation**] Blood and sweat have one and the same source; Blood and sweat share the same source; Blood and sweat share the same origin; blood and sweat being of the same source

[**Standard Translation**] Blood and sweat are of the same origin.

Citations

- Little perspiration is seen in patients with excessive hemorrhage, and blood deficiency is found in patients with profuse sweating. (*Spiritual Pivot*)
- Blood and sweat are of the same origin and should not be damaged simultaneously. (*The Concise Book of Cold Damage*)

16. QÌ ZHǓ XÙZHĪ 气主煦之

Qi Warms the Body

Qi generates heat and warms the human body. Its warming function is mainly embodied in the following aspects. First, qi generates heat and maintains relatively constant body temperature. Qi is the material basis of heat production in the body. It continuously generates heat in its movement to warm the body. Besides, defense qi controls the opening and closing of sweat pores and regulates body temperature by regulating the excretion of sweat. Second, qi warms the zang-fu organs, meridians, and other tissues to ensure their physiological functions. Third, qi maintains the circulation of liquid substances such as essence, blood, and body fluids. Weakened warming function of qi and reduced heat production may cause such pathological changes as low body temperature, cold limbs, visceral dysfunction, and unsmooth circulation of essence, blood, and body fluids.

[**Previous Translation**] Qi dominates warmth
[**Current Translation**] Warming function of qi; qi warming body; qi governing warmth
[**Standard Translation**] Qi warms the body.

Citations

- Qi warms the human body, while blood nourishes and moistens it. (*Canon of Difficult Issues*)
- Qi warming the body means qi produces heat to "steam" human skin and muscles. (*Differentiating the Meaning of "Canon of Difficult Issues"*)
- Qi warms the human body. Through qi the whole body is warmed and nourished. (*Tests of All Subjects by Imperial Medical Bureau*)

17. XUÈ ZHǓ RÚZHĪ 血主濡之

Blood Nourishes and Moistens the Body

Blood, composed of nutrient qi and body fluids, provides nutrients and moisture to the human body. Nutrient qi is the refined essence transformed from the essence of food and drinks; body fluids are to moisten the whole body. Therefore, the primary function of blood is nourishing and moistening. Blood circulates in the blood vessels throughout the body, reaching the zang-fu organs, skin, muscles, tendons, and vessels, constantly nourishing and moistening them to maintain their normal physiological functions and ensure life activities. Reddish complexion, clear vision, strong muscles, bones, and tendons, lustrous skin and hair, and quick perception as well as flexibility in physical movement are evidences of blood sufficiency and the normal functioning of blood in nourishing and moistening. Otherwise, sallow complexion, blurred vision, pale lips and nails, dry hair and skin, muscle wasting, flaccidity of tendons and muscles, limb numbness, inflexibility in physical movement, and thready pulse may occur.

[**Previous Translation**] Blood dominates nourishment; Blood dominates moisture and nourishment
[**Current Translation**] Blood serving nutritive function; Blood is responsible for moistening and nourishment; blood being responsible for nurturing body; blood governing moisture and nourishment
[**Standard Translation**] Blood nourishes and moistens the body.

Citations

- Qi warms the human body, while blood nourishes and moistens it. (*Canon of Difficult Issues*)
- Blood nourishing and moistening the human body means blood can moisten bones and tendons, lubricate joints, and nourish the zang-fu organs. (*Differentiating the Meaning of "Canon of Difficult Issues"*)
- Blood has the function of nourishing and moistening the human body. In cases of blood deficiency, spasm of tendons may occur due to the failure of blood to nourish them. (*Annotated "Treatise on Cold Damage"*)

18. QÌ WÉI XUÈ SHUÀI 气为血帅

Qi Is the Commander of Blood

Qi can generate, promote, and control blood, which is generally described as "qi being the commander of blood." First, qi generates blood, that is, qi is involved in and promotes the generation of blood. When qi is abundant, blood will be sufficient. When qi is weak, blood will be deficient. Prolonged qi deficiency often causes insufficient generation of blood and therefore blood-deficiency pattern occurs. Second, qi promotes blood circulation, that is, qi is the driving force of blood circulation. As qi flows, blood flows. When qi stops, blood flow stops. If qi is weak or stagnates, unsmooth or sluggish flow of blood or even blood stasis may occur. If there is qi disorder with abnormal ascending, descending, exiting, or entering, blood circulation will be affected, and bleeding may occur as a result of abnormal blood flow following the adverse flow of qi or the sinking of qi. Third, qi contains blood. Qi has the function of controlling blood to flow in the vessels and preventing it from escaping out of the vessels. In the case of qi deficiency with weakened controlling function, hemorrhagic diseases may occur such as hematuria, hemafecia, metrorrhagia, metrostaxis, and purpura, which is described as deficient qi failing to control blood.

[**Previous Translation**] Vital energy as the commander of blood; "QI" (VITAL ENERGY) AS THE COMMANDER OF BLOOD; vital energy as the commander of blood; Qi is the commander of blood; Qi acts as the commander of Blood

[**Current Translation**] Qi as the commander of blood; qi being (the) commander of blood; Qi is the commander of blood; qi commanding blood

[**Standard Translation**] Qi is the commander of blood.

Citations

- Qi is the commander of blood; therefore, qi should be regulated before menstrual regulation. (*A Summary of Gynecology*)
- In the case of bleeding due to the adverse flow of qi, follow Master Miao's approach that qi is the commander of blood, using *suzi* (*Fructus Perillae*, perilla fruit), *yujin* (*Radix Curcumae*, curcuma root), *sangye* (*Folium Mori*, mulberry leaf), *danpi* (*Cortex Moutan Radicis*, moutan bark), *jiangxiang* (*Lignum Dalbergiae Odorifera*, dalbergia wood), and *chuanbei* (*Bulbus Fritillariae Cirrhosae*, Sichuan fritillary bulb) to treat it. (*Case Records: A Guide to Clinical Practice*)

19. XUÈ WÉI QÌ MǓ 血为气母

Blood Is the Mother of Qi

Blood can generate and carry qi, which is generally described as "blood being the mother of qi." First, blood generates qi. Blood circulates all over the body, continuously providing nutrition for the generation and functional activities of qi to maintain its normal physiological function.

Therefore, qi is vigorous when blood is abundant and qi becomes weak when blood is deficient. Second, blood is the carrier of qi, a vehicle to bring qi to the whole body. Qi pertains to yang and is dynamic; blood pertains to yin and is static. Therefore, qi must depend on tangible blood for normal circulation. Otherwise, qi will float and scatter if blood fails to carry qi and qi has nothing to depend on. For example, in patients with massive hemorrhage, qi will collapse, resulting in a deadly disease known as qi desertion following blood loss; or qi stagnation may occur when there is obstruction in blood circulation.

[**Previous Translation**] Blood as the mother of vital energy; BLOOD IS THE MOTHER OF QI (VITAL ENERGY); Blood is the mother of qi; blood being the mother of qi; Blood is the material foundation of Qi
[**Current Translation**] Blood being (the) mother of qi; Blood is the mother of qi
[**Standard Translation**] Blood is the mother of qi.

Citations

• Blood carries qi, and qi transports blood. (*Treatise on Blood Syndromes*)
• Qi and blood guard each other, so they are inseparable. (*A Close Examination of the Precious Classic on Ophthalmology*)

20. SHÉNJĪ QÌLÌ 神机气立

Vital Activity and Qi Configuration

Vital activity is the foundation of life. It embodies the mechanism of governing and regulating life activities. Qi configuration, meaning qi movement in nature, is the condition on which life is sustained. These two concepts, though relatively independent, are closely related. They jointly reveal the overall connection between the generating and transforming activities of a living organism and its internal and external environment.

Vital activity, relative to qi configuration, mainly refers to the regulation and control of qi movement in the human body and is the internal basis of life. By means of organized and purposeful self-regulation and movement, it ensures a steady state of the internal environment (homeostasis) and maintains the coordination of the internal and the external environments of a human body with the assistance of qi configuration.

Qi configuration mainly refers to the exchange and transformation of "qi" between the living organism and the natural environment, that is, the exchange of substance, energy, and information. It is the condition on which the organism depends for survival and the manifestation of the regulation and control of vital activity. Vital activity and qi configuration complement each other to maintain the normal life activities of the living body.

[**Previous Translation**] Vital activity; mysterious mechanism (神机)
[**Current Translation**] Vital activity; mysterious mechanism; SPIRITUAL MECHANISM (神机); vital activity and qi configuration; shenji (magic mechanism) (神机); qili (origination of qi) (气立)
[**Standard Translation**] Vital activity and qi configuration

Citations

- What originates from the interior of creatures is called vital activity. Generation and transformation will stop when the vitality is gone. What originates from the exterior of things is called qi configuration. Generation and transformation will cease if qi activity stops. (*Plain Conversation*)
- When qi ceases exiting and entering, vital activities shall vanish; when qi ceases ascending and descending, qi configuration shall perish. (*Plain Conversation*)
- With blood and qi, animals have their vitality rooted in the interior of the body with spirit dominating the life, which is called vital activity.... On the part of plants and minerals, their vitality is rooted in the exterior with qi dominating the growth, which is called qi configuration. (*Classified Classics*)

21. JĪNGMÀI 经脉

① *Meridian* ② *Normal Pulse*

The term *jingmai* (in most cases translated as meridians) refers to the trunk routes in the meridian system. Meridians are the main pathways for the flow of qi and blood as well as the conduction of sensations and are classified into three categories: twelve (regular) meridians, eight extra meridians, and twelve divergent meridians. The twelve meridians, also called twelve principal meridians, are directly connected with the zang-fu organs. They begin, connect, and end at particular points, running along fixed routes in particular directions. The eight extra meridians, however, unlike the twelve principal meridians, do not pertain to any zang-fu organs and they are not exterior-interiorly related. They have the effects of governing, coordinating, and regulating qi and blood in the twelve meridians. The twelve divergent meridians are the branches which derive from, enter, leave, and join the twelve principal meridians. They strengthen the connection between the exterior-interiorly paired meridians and supplement the twelve principal meridians. As pulse diagnosis constitutes a major part of the origins of meridian theory, *jingmai* may also be used in Chinese medical classics to refer to normal pulse manifestation, as opposed to *bing-mai* (morbid pulse).

[**Previous Translation**] Meridian and vessels; meridian; channels and vessels; meridians; channels; CHANNEL; jing-mai (the channels); channel vessel

[**Current Translation**] Meridians; channel; main meridian; meridian

[**Standard Translation**] ① Meridian ② Normal pulse

Citations

- Meridians are the pathways through which qi and blood flow as well as yin and yang aspects are transported to nourish the body, moisten tendons and bones, and lubricate joints. (*Spiritual Pivot*)
- The twelve meridians run deep in the muscular interstice and therefore are invisible. (*Spiritual Pivot*)
- Only when one has fully understood the normal pulse can he/she know what a morbid pulse is. (*Plain Conversation*)

22. LUÒMÀI 络脉

Collateral

Collaterals are the branches of meridians, forming an intricate reticulated network throughout the body. They are further divided into divergent and tertiary collaterals according to sizes. Divergent collaterals, also called "fifteen divergent collaterals," are the larger and major collaterals, which can strengthen the connection between the exterior-interiorly paired meridians on the body surface. Tertiary collaterals are further divisions of these collaterals, extending from linear connection to surface diffusion, to further strengthen the connection at tissue level and promote the infusion of qi and blood.

From the perspective of yin-yang property, there are yin collaterals and yang collaterals. Yin collaterals run downward and are in the interior, connecting with the zang-organs. Yang collaterals go upward and are in the exterior, connecting with the fu-organs. From the perspective of qi and blood, there are qi collaterals and blood collaterals. Qi collaterals are featured by qi flow while blood collaterals by blood flow. From the perspective of zang-fu organs, different names are assigned to collaterals according to their locations. For example, there are zang collateral, heart collateral, lung collateral, brain collateral, stomach collateral, and so on. Collaterals are primarily responsible for supplying tissues with qi and blood, bringing their nourishing and moistening effects into play.

[**Previous Translation**] Collaterals and subcollaterals; collateral; collaterals; collateral vessel; luo-mai (the collateral channels); network vessel
[**Current Translation**] Collaterals; network vessel; collateral (meridian); collateral
[**Standard Translation**] Collateral

Citations

- All vessels on the surface and visible to the eyes are collaterals. (*Spiritual Pivot*)
- In terms of diagnosis of the collaterals, blueness of the vessels indicates cold stagnation with pain, while redness of the vessels indicates heat. (*Spiritual Pivot*)
- When wine is ingested into the stomach, the collaterals will be filled with blood. The meridians, however, will be empty. (*Plain Conversation*)

23. LIÙYÍN 六淫

Six Excesses

Six excesses refer to the six exogenous pathogens including wind, cold, summer-heat, dampness, dryness, and fire. Generally, six excesses are closely related to six qi which refers to the normal climatic variations in nature (wind, cold, summer-heat, dampness, dryness, and fire/heat). Normal climatic changes are not pathogenic. Nevertheless, when they become unusual, that is, excessive or deficient, unseasonable, or sudden and violent, to the extent that the human body cannot adapt to the changes, diseases would then arise. In such cases, six qi becomes six excesses.

Six excesses are virtually the etiological model established for determining the causes of diseases by drawing an analogy between the characteristics of the climatic variations in nature (wind, cold, summer-heat, dampness, dryness, and fire) and clinical manifestations in the human body. They are the synthesis and summary of six etiological factors in accordance with the patterns identified in humans, a comprehensive functional model of exogenous pathogens based on overall physical responses to different causes to figure out responses for various situations.

[**Previous Translation**] Six exopathogens; six exogenous pathogenic factors; six climatic evils; SIX CLIMATIC EXOPATHOGENS; six excesses
[**Current Translation**] Six climate conditions in excess as pathogenic factors; six excesses; adverse environmental conditions of wind, cold, dryness, dampness, fire, and summer-heat
[**Standard Translation**] six excesses

Citations

- Six excesses refer to six kinds of pathogenic factors, namely, cold, summer-heat, dryness, dampness, wind, and fire. (*Discussion of Pathology Based on Triple Etiology Doctrine*)
- Third, six excesses refer to the exogenous pathogens including wind, cold, summer-heat, dampness, dryness, and fire that may invade the human body and cause diseases. (*Tests of All Subjects by Imperial Medical Bureau*)

- Those who are adversely affected by six excesses should first have their qi regulated and then be treated individually according to the identified pathogenic factor. (*Precepts for Physicians*)

24. QĪQÍNG 七情

Seven Emotions

The term refers to seven emotional activities: joy, anger, anxiety, over-thinking, sorrow, fear, and fright. They are the emotional responses to external stimuli. In most cases, they would not cause or trigger diseases. Only when they become excessive in intensity or duration, exceeding the psychological and physiological adaptability of a human being, would essential qi of the zang-fu organs be impaired and functional disorders arise. Diseases would occur when healthy qi is deficient, zang-fu organs' essential qi is consumed, and the human body's adaptability to emotional stimuli is lowered. Usually two or more emotions are interlaced to cause diseases, harming the five zang-organs, disturbing qi movement, and leading to psychological conditions that are oftentimes complicated to treat.

[**Previous Translation**] Seven modes of emotion; seven emotions; seven affects
[**Current Translation**] Seven emotions; seven affects
[**Standard Translation**] Seven emotions

Citations

- Seven emotions refer to joy, anger, anxiety, over-thinking, sorrow, fear, and fright.... As part of human characteristics, seven emotions are endogenous factors that may cause diseases. They would adversely affect people's health when they are restrained in zang-fu organs and manifest themselves in the exterior. (*Discussion of Pathology Based on Triple Etiology Doctrine*)
- Infertility in women may result from the impairment of thorough-fare vessel and conception vessel caused by six excesses and/or excess of seven emotions. (*Complete Effective Prescriptions for Women's Diseases*)

- There are six excesses in nature, namely, wind, cold, summer-heat, dampness, dryness, and fire, while people may suffer internal impairment by seven emotions, namely, joy, anger, anxiety, over-thinking, sorrow, fear, and fright. (*Revealing the Mystery of the Origin of Eye Diseases*)

25. ZHÈNGQÌ 正气

Healthy Qi

The term refers to the normal functional activities of life substances (essence, qi, blood, fluids, etc.) and structures (zang-fu organs, meridians, etc.) of the human body as well as the capability to maintain health including self-regulation, adaptation to the environment, disease resistance, prevention, self-healing, and recovery. The abundance of healthy qi depends on the following conditions: (1) intact structures of tissues, zang-fu organs, meridians, and so on; (2) sufficient supply of life substances including essence, qi, blood, and fluids; (3) normal function and interaction of all life activities. Among them, essence, qi, blood, and fluids are the material basis of all functional activities, and their abundance ensures the normal function and coordination between tissues and organs as well as a prosperous healthy qi. As essence, qi, blood, and fluids are the decisive factors for the condition of healthy qi, their conditions are often viewed as important bases for determining the status of healthy qi.

[**Previous Translation**] Healthy qi; vital qi; genuine qi; zheng qi (the primordial principle); right qi
[**Current Translation**] Vital-qi; right qi; healthy qi; normal qi; body resistance; genuine qi
[**Standard Translation**] Healthy qi

Citations

- In terms of the five kinds of pestilence… if there is no infection when the five kinds of pestilence occur, it is because healthy qi is abundant in the body and pathogenic qi has no way to invade. (*Plain Conversation*)

- The pulse manifestations are equal at *cun* (寸), *guan* (关), and *chi* (尺), the three sections over the radial artery, reflecting that healthy qi is in harmony. In such cases, although pathogenic qi is not eliminated, what damage will there be? (*Annotated "Treatise on Cold Damage"*)
- Pathogenic wind and cold invade the body due to the weakness of zang-fu organs, causing the fight between healthy qi and pathogenic qi, resulting in abdominal pain. (*Treatise on the Origins and Manifestations of Various Diseases*)

26. XIÉQÌ 邪气

Pathogenic Qi

The term refers to all kinds of pathogenic factors, including those in the external environment and those inside the body. Examples are six excesses, pestilential qi, excess of seven emotions, dietary irregularities, lack of exercises or excessive labor, trauma, insect bites or animal injuries, parasites, water dampness, phlegm retention, static blood, and stones. Pathogenic qi may bring the following harms to the human body: (1) physiological abnormalities leading to yin-yang imbalance, functional disorders of zang-fu organs and meridians, and metabolic and functional disorders of essence, qi, blood, fluids; (2) damaging the integrity of zang-fu organs and tissues; (3) changing an individual's constitution and altering the predisposition to disease; and (4) impairing the body's resistance to disease and the ability to heal on its own.

[**Previous Translation**] Pathogenic factors; evils; PATHOGENIC QI; xie (evil) qi; evil qi
[**Current Translation**] Pathogenic factors; evil qi; pathogenic factor; pathogen; the evil qi
[**Standard Translation**] Pathogenic qi

Citations

- When pathogenic qi attacks the skin and hair, it enters the lung to which the skin and hair pertain. (*Plain Conversation*)

- The occurrence of disease is not inherent, but caused by pathogenic qi resulting from either external invasion or internal transformation. (*Confucians' Duties to Their Parents*)
- When pulse manifestation is found to correspond to the four seasons, it indicates abundance of healthy qi in the body. Though invaded by pathogenic qi, one can have pathogens relieved with slight spontaneous sweating. (*Annotated "Treatise on Cold Damage"*)

27. NÙ ZÉ QÌSHÀNg 怒则气上

Rage Drives Qi Upward

Rage leads to the adverse flow of liver qi or blood, making qi and blood flow upward. Liver is the organ that pertains to wind and wood, which stores tangible blood and promotes the flow of intangible qi. Anger is the emotion associated with the liver. Persistent excessive anger can make liver qi disperse excessively, leading to the upward counterflow of liver qi or even blood. Clinical manifestations include distending headache, redness of face and eyes, vexation, irritability, and even hematemesis, or syncope. Long-term depression and anger may also bring the failure of the liver to disperse qi, causing liver qi stagnation characterized by distending pain in the chest, hypochondria, breasts, and lower abdomen, as well as preference for deep sighing and so on. If liver qi subjugates the spleen, abdominal pain and diarrhea may occur.

[**Previous Translation**] Anger causes the Qi (vital energy) of the liver to go perversely upward; anger arousing ascent of qi; ANGER MAY LEAD TO THE ABNORMAL RISING OF VITAL ENERGY; Rage causes the qi (of the liver) to flow adversely upward; Abnormal rising of vital energy due to anger; Anger may lead to the abnormal rising of vital energy; Rage causes adverse flow of liver Qi

[**Current Translation**] Adverse flow of the liver-qi caused by rage; Rage drives qi upward; rage causing adverse flow of liver Qi to go adversely upward; Rage causing qi to flow adversely upward; anger causes qi to rise; rage causing qi rising; Rages drives qi upward

[**Standard Translation**] Rage drives qi upward.

Citations

- Rage drives qi upward... Excessive anger leads to the adverse flow of qi, or even hematemesis and *sunxie* (diarrhea with indigested food). Therefore, "qi flows upwards." (*Plain Conversation*)
- Rage disturbs yang qi and drives qi and blood upward to stagnate in the head, eventually resulting in syncope. (*Plain Conversation*)
- Being fiery and forthright, these kinds of people tend to get angry easily. When they get angry, qi will flow adversely upward and accumulate in the chest, causing unsmooth flow of qi and blood. (*Spiritual Pivot*)

28. SĪ ZÉ QÌJIÉ 思则气结

Over-thinking Binds Qi

Over-thinking can cause unsmooth flow of qi. Thought or thinking is the emotion associated with the spleen. Over-thinking may result in qi stagnation in the spleen and the stomach, inadequate ascending and descending of qi, and the failure of transportation and transformation. Its manifestations include poor appetite, abdominal distension, and diarrhea. Over time, it will lead to insufficient production of qi and blood, manifested as dizziness, fatigue, muscle wasting, and so on. In addition, over-thinking may consume heart blood, deprive the heart spirit of nourishment, and cause such symptoms as palpitations, insomnia, and dream-disturbed sleep.

[**Previous Translation**] Mental anxiety makes the Qi (vital energy) of the spleen depressed; worry causing stagnation of qi; ANXIETY MAY LEAD TO STAGNATION OF VITAL ENERGY; Anxiety makes the qi (of the spleen) depressed; Anxiety makes qi depressed; anxiety making qi depressed; Over-thinking may lead to the depression of vital energy; the depression of the vital energy caused by over-thinking; anxiety making Qi depressed; anxiety makes Qi depressed; Anxiety making Qi stagnation

[**Current Translation**] Anxiety making qi depressed; anxiety causing qi stagnation; Anxiety makes qi depressed; Thought causes qi to bind; pensiveness causing qi to stagnation; pensiveness generating qi stuckness

[**Standard Translation**] Over-thinking binds qi.

Citations

- Over-thinking causes qi to bind… Excessive thinking leads to the concentration of mind and spirit on a particular issue so that healthy qi is retained and fails to circulate properly. Therefore, "qi binds." (*Plain Conversation*)
- Over-thinking causes qi to bind. Qi stagnates in the heart, and the spleen may be affected. (*Jingyue's Complete Works*)

29. XǏ ZÉ QÌHUǍN 喜则气缓

Excessive Joy Slackens Qi

Excessive joy slackens heart qi. Joy is the emotion associated with the heart and is a type of beneficial emotional response. Moderate joy can regulate the flow of qi and blood, make nutrient qi and defense qi unobstructed, and maintain ease of mind and a relaxed mood, relieving mental tension. However, excessive joy can easily slacken heart qi. In severe cases, collapse of heart qi, absent-mindedness, restlessness, inattention, insomnia, and even hysterical laughing, incoherent speech, and other abnormal behaviors may occur. As stated in the "Basic State of Spirit" of *Spiritual Pivot*, "excessive joy and happiness cause heart qi to disperse and spirit is no longer stored."

[**Previous Translation**] Joy inducing sluggishness of qi; Over joy may lead to the sluggishness of vital energy; EXCESSIVE JOY MAKES THE QI (OF THE HEART) SLUGGISH; An excess of joy may lead to the sluggishness of vital energy; Joy induces sluggishness of qi; joy inducing sluggishness of qi; Excessive Joy inducing relaxation of qi; excessive joy brings about descent of Qi.

[**Current Translation**] Over joy relaxing qi; excessive joy inducing relaxation of qi; excessive joy relaxing Qi (of heart); Joy causes qi to slacken; over-joy causing qi to slacken; Over-joy leads to sluggishness of heart qi

[**Standard Translation**] Excessive joy slackens qi.

Citations

- Excessive joy slackens qi... Moderate joy and happiness lead to harmony of qi, ease of mind, and smooth flow of nutrient qi and defense qi. Over-joy, nevertheless, makes qi slacken and dissipate. (*Plain Conversation*)
- Joy and happiness make qi and will harmonious and well-regulated so that disease will not arise. However, excessive joy will make heart qi dissipate and unable to maintain inside, causing hysterical laughing and failure of qi to astringe. In severe cases, manic symptoms may occur. (*Stepping Stones for Medicine*)
- The heart stores spirit and corresponds to joy in emotion. Excessive joy makes heart qi slacken and dissipate so that heart-qi deficiency and loss of mind can be found. Sour foods are advised to take to astringe heart qi. (*Renewed Materia Medica*)

30. BĒI ZÉ QÌXIĀO 悲则气消

Excessive Sorrow Exhausts Qi

Excessive sorrow consumes lung qi because sorrow is the emotion associated with the lung. Excessive sorrow dissipates healthy qi, especially lung qi, which causes its dysfunction of ascending, dispersing, purifying, and descending. Clinical manifestations include shortness of breath, no desire to speak, low voice and faint breathing, lassitude, lack of strength, low spirit, susceptibility to colds, and so on.

[**Previous Translation**] Excessive sorrow dissipating qi; Sorrow may lead to the consumption of vital energy; SORROW MAKES THE QI (OF THE LUNG) CONSUMED; excessive sorrow dissipating qi; Excessive sorrow leads to consumption of qi; Sadness may lead to the consumption of vital energy; excessive sorrow leading to consumption of qi; Excessive sadness leads to Qi consumption

[**Current Translation**] Excessive sorrow resulting in consumption of qi; qi consumption due to grief; Sorrow makes the qi consumed; excessive sorrow leading to consumption Qi; Sorrow causes qi to disperse; sorrow causing qi consumption; lung qi consumption due to over-grief

[**Standard Translation**] Excessive sorrow exhausts qi.

Citations

- Sorrow may exhaust qi.... Excessive sorrow may lead to the contraction of the heart and the expansion of the lung, causing the failure of the upper energizer to disperse qi and the failure of nutrient qi and defense qi to be distributed. Therefore, qi is restrained and transformed into heat and the heat-qi in the interior impairs healthy qi; hence "qi is exhausted." (*Plain Conversation*)
- Excessive sorrow exhausts qi, which leads to empty pulse. (*The A-B Classic of Acupuncture and Moxibustion*)
- Excessive sorrow exhausts qi. If one's will and intents are suppressed by frustration, one will feel depressed and qi will be dissipated. (*Stepping Stones for Medicine*)

31. KŎNG ZÉ QÌXIÀ 恐则气下

Excessive Fear Drives Qi Downward

Excessive fear can lead to insecurity and sinking of kidney qi because fear is the emotion associated with the kidney. Being subject to sudden fright or persistent fear can impair the kidney, causing kidney qi to flow downward and become unconsolidated, and lead to the sinking and exhaustion of essential qi. Clinical manifestations include fecal and urinary incontinence, seminal emission, menstrual disorders, or increased leucorrhea. As a result of the loss of essential qi, soreness and weakness of the lower back and knee, weakness of both feet, and other symptoms may occur.

[**Previous Translation**] Fear causes the Qi (vital energy) of the kidney to sink; fear causing descent of qi; TERROR MAY LEAD TO THE COLLAPSE OF VITAL ENERGY; Fear causes the qi (of the kidney) to sink; Fear causes descent of qi; Fright causes sinking of qi;Terror may lead to the abnormal falling of vital energy; Fear leads to sinking of Qi; Fear Causing Sinking of Kidney-qi

[**Current Translation**] Fright causing sinking of qi; Fear causes qi to sink; Terror may lead to the sinking of qi; fear causing qi sinking; Fear causes qi sinking

[**Standard Translation**] Excessive fear drives qi downward.

Citations

- Excessive fear drives qi downward.... Excessive fear may lead to the sinking of essential qi, making the kidney unable to coordinate with the heart and the lung, causing qi obstruction of the upper energizer, and leading to the return of qi and distension of the lower energizer. Therefore, qi is driven downward. (*Plain Conversation*)
- Excessive fear without relief will impair essence, and the impairment of essence will cause soreness and weakness of bones, flaccidity, and syncope, accompanied with habitual seminal emission in most cases. (*Spiritual Pivot*)
- Excessive fright causes derangement of qi and excessive fear causes sinking of qi. The liver and the kidney will inevitably be impaired. (*Jingyue's Complete Works*)

32. JĪNG ZÉ QÌLUÀN 惊则气乱

Excessive Fright Deranges Qi

Sudden fear or fright may cause disorder of heart qi, which then leads to disharmony between qi and blood. Fright is one's response to a sudden event, for example, upon witnessing something unusual or being startled suddenly. It is a protective psychological mechanism for human beings to deal with negative external stimuli. Fright can cause disorder of qi movement, leading to deranged qi flow and abnormal mental states. Clinical manifestations include palpitation, restlessness, panic, insomnia, and being easily startled. Some patients may even have manic symptoms such as incoherent speech, fanatic crying and laughing, manic raving, and agitation.

[**Previous Translation**] Fright causing disturbances of qi; Terror may lead to disorder of vital energy; FRIGHT LEADS TO DISTURBANCE OF QI; Excessive fright leads to disturbance of Qi

[**Current Translation**] Disturbance of the flow of qi caused by fright; fright disturbing qi; fright disrupting qi; fright causing disorder of qi; qi disorder due to terror

[**Standard Translation**] Excessive fright deranges qi.

Citations

- Excessive fright causes derangement of qi.... Sudden fear or fright leads to palpitation, mental distraction, and hesitation. Therefore, qi is deranged. (*Plain Conversation*)
- Fright diarrhea occurs as the heart is startled. Fright causes derangement of qi, leading to the obstruction of heart qi and the inflow of water-fluid to intestines, which then causes diarrhea. (*Symptoms, Causes, Pulses, and Treatments*)
- Fright is derived from external stimuli. It may cause derangement of qi. Therefore, the patient's pulse feels restless. (*Extensive Annotations on "Essential Prescriptions of the Golden Cabinet"*)

33. HÁN ZÉ QÌSHŌU 寒则气收

Excessive Cold Causes Qi to Contract

Pathogenic cold invades the body and causes qi to contract, leading to the contraction and spasm of interstices, meridians, tendons, and vessels. Cold-induced diseases are characterized by contraction. When pathogenic cold invades the surface of the skin and muscles, it closes the pores and muscular interstices, thus constraining the defensive yang from dispersion. Clinical manifestations include a version to cold, fever, and absence of sweat. When cold invades the blood vessels, stagnation of qi and blood and spasm of blood vessels may occur, which may be manifested as headache and pain in the body with tight pulse. When cold invades meridians and joints, contraction and spasm of joints may arise, which can be manifested as inhibited bending and stretching or having cold and numb joints.

[**Previous Translation**] Cold induces contraction; Cold-evil renders the energy sluggish; COLD CAUSES CONTRACTION

[**Current Translation**] Cold renders yang-qi sluggish; Cold makes qi compact; cold astringing qi; cold contracting qi; cold causing qi to contract

[**Standard Translation**] Excessive cold causes qi to contract.

Citations

- Excessive cold causes qi to contract.... Excessive cold leads to closure of muscular interstices and obstruction of qi flow. Therefore, "qi contracts." (*Plain Conversation*)
- The pathogenesis that excessive cold causes qi to contract is perhaps as follows: when human body is affected by pathogenetic cold, muscular interstices would be closed, and then defense qi would fail to reach the superficial part of the body. As a result, the qi of the zang-fu organs would be astringed inside. (*Annotations and Commentary of Plain Conversation in Yellow Emperor's Internal Canon of Medicine*)
- Excessive cold causes qi to contract. Its treatment requires the use of pungent herbals to disperse qi and sweet medicines to relieve it. (*Detailed Explanation of the Jade Pivot*)

34. JIŎNG ZÉ QÌXIÈ 炅则气泄

Excessive Heat Causes Discharge of Qi

Pathogenic summer-heat could give rise to the opening of muscular interstices and the discharge of healthy qi. Characterized by ascent and dispersion, pathogenic summer-heat forces fluids to discharge from opened pores. Along with the loss of fluids, qi is also discharged as fluids carry qi. Clinically, it can be manifested as fluid consumption and qi deficiency. The former includes thirst with a desire for drinks and scanty dark-colored urine, while the latter includes shortness of breath and fatigue. When qi and fluids are exhausted in severe cases, sudden fainting and unconsciousness may occur due to the lack of nourishment in clear orifices.

[**Previous Translation**] Fever leading to consumption of vital energy; heat leads to discharge of qi

[**Current Translation**] HEAT CONSUMES VITAL ENERGY; Heat leads to discharge of qi; Heat makes qi dispersed; fever resulting in dissipation of the yang principle; overheat causing qi leakage

[**Standard Translation**] Excessive heat causes discharge of qi.

Citations

- Excessive heat causes discharge of qi.... Excessive summer-heat makes muscular interstices open, brings smooth flow of nutrient qi and defense qi, and induces profuse sweating. Qi will be discharged along with perspiration; hence "qi is discharged." (*Plain Conversation*)
- Excessive heat causes discharge of qi. Now pathogenic summer-heat invades defense qi, and fever and spontaneous sweat can be examined. *Huangqi* (*Radix Astragali*, astragalus root), which supplements qi with sweet-warm, should be used as monarch drug. (*Treatise on the Spleen and Stomach*)

35. LÁO ZÉ QÌHÀO 劳则气耗

Overexertion Consumes Qi

Overexertion usually causes consumption of healthy qi. Overexertion leads to excessive panting and sweating. Excessive panting consumes lung qi, while over-sweating may lead to deficiency of healthy qi as qi could be discharged along with the loss of fluids. Consumption of healthy qi, especially lung qi and spleen qi, is thus developed. Clinically, it is often manifested as shortness of breath, no desire to speak, lassitude, lack of strength, and fatigue in the extremities.

[**Previous Translation**] Overexertion may lead to consumption of vital energy; overexertion leading to consumption of qi

[**Current Translation**] OVER-EXERTION LEADING TO QI EXHAUSTION; strain makes qi consumed; overstrain leading to consumption of qi; overexertion leading to qi consumption; overexertion causing loss of qi; qi exhaustion due to extreme tiredness

[**Standard Translation**] Overexertion consumes qi.

Citations

- Overexertion consumes qi.... It leads to panting, sweating, and leakage of healthy qi in the interior and exterior of the human body. Therefore, "qi is consumed." (*Plain Conversation*)
- The reason why overexertion causes consumption of qi is that overexertion will disturb qi movement and lead to panting and sweating. Panting causes qi in the interior to disperse, while sweating causes qi to disperse outside. As a result, qi is consumed and dissipated. (*Annotations and Commentary* of *Plain Conversation in Yellow Emperor's Internal Canon of Medicine*)
- Perhaps overexertion causes consumption of qi and lung qi is then impaired, which leads to hoarseness. (*Shishan's Case Records*)

36. XIÉZHÈNG SHÈNGSHUĀI 邪正盛衰

Exuberance and Debilitation of Pathogenic Qi and Healthy Qi

The term refers to the change in strength (i.e., exuberance and debilitation) of healthy qi and pathogenic qi in their combat as diseases develop. Healthy qi may be impaired when pathogenic qi invades the body, but on the other hand, healthy qi can defend and expel pathogens. The tendency and the result of the combat will not only determine the occurrence of diseases, but affect the development, prognosis, and excess/deficiency of the condition. In the combat, if both healthy qi and pathogenic qi are exuberant, the fight will be fierce, and excess patterns may occur in most cases; if both healthy qi and pathogenic qi are debilitated, deficiency patterns may arise in most cases; if pathogenic qi is exuberant and healthy qi is debilitated, deficiency-excess complex patterns may be found in most cases.

[**Previous Translation**] Prosperity and decline of the evil and the genuine; excess and weakness of evil and vital qi; EXUBERANCE AND DEBILITATION

[**Current Translation**] Exuberance and decline of pathogenic factors and healthy qi; preponderance and decline; excess and decline; exuberance and debilitation

[**Standard Translation**] Exuberance and debilitation of pathogenic qi and healthy qi

Citations

- Even when there are accumulations in the excess pattern, drastic medicinals cannot be overused, not to mention when there are accumulations in the deficiency pattern. This is one consideration in the treatment of accumulation. The exuberance and debilitation of healthy qi and pathogenic qi should be evaluated meticulously. (*Jingyue's Complete Works*)
- Generation, restriction, over-restriction, and counter-restriction among the five elements and pulse manifestation in terms of exuberance and debilitation of pathogenic qi and healthy qi should be evaluated before treatment. (*Collection of Experience on Cold Damage*)
- If one fails to understand the changes in dominant qi of the year, and only considers whether it is cold or heat, one cannot differentiate exuberance and debilitation of pathogenic qi and healthy qi. (*Effective Use of Established Formulas*)

37. ZHĒNSHÍ JIǍXŪ 真实假虚

True Excess with Pseudo-deficiency

The term refers to the clinical situation where the nature of a disease is excess, but instead, deficiency is manifested in disguise. It is caused by internal accumulation of hyperactive pathogenic qi obstructing meridians and restraining qi and blood from reaching outside. The pattern is also known as the "occurrence of deficiency manifestations in extreme excess." For example, when heat binds in the stomach and the intestines as in the pattern of intense interior heat, excess heat symptoms can be manifested as constipation, abdominal pain with rigidity and fullness, or even delirium. On the other hand, as yang qi is blocked inside and unable to disperse, pseudo-deficiency cold symptoms may occur such as pale complexion, reversal cold of the extremities, and lassitude.

[**Previous Translation**] Asthenia-syndrome in appearance but sthenia-syndrome in nature; excess syndrome with pseudo-deficiency; REAL EXCESS WITH PSEUDO-DEFICIENCY

[**Current Translation**] Syndrome of excess type with pseudo-deficiency symptoms; sthenia syndrome with pseudo-asthenia symptoms; true

sthenia and false asthenia syndrome; true excess and false deficiency syndrome; excess syndrome with pseudo-deficiency symptoms; true excess with false deficiency; excess syndrome with pseudo-deficiency
[**Standard Translation**] True excess with pseudo-deficiency

Citations

- One cannot be so sure that the pattern of true excess with pseudo-deficiency manifestations does not exist. For instance, endogenous pathogenetic cold or food accumulation causes qi stagnation and may lead to acute pain in the heart and the abdomen with deep, hidden, abrupt or knotted pulse. It is caused by pathogenic qi blocking meridians. Although pulse manifestations may indicate deficiency, there must be such excess symptoms as pain and distension. This is the pulse manifestation of pseudo-deficiency, but not deficiency pattern in nature. (*Jingyue's Complete Works*)
- One cannot be so sure that the pattern of true excess with pseudo-deficiency manifestations does not exist. While mild diseases should be treated in accordance with symptoms, serious diseases must be treated in accordance with pulse manifestation. This is the appropriate method. (*Interpretation on Pulses*)

38. ZHĒNXŪ JIǍSHÍ 真虚假实

True Deficiency with Pseudo-excess

The term refers to the clinical condition of a patient whose disease is deficiency in nature, but instead, excess is manifested in disguise. The phenomenon is mainly attributable to the deficiency of healthy qi in the zang-fu organs and meridians, leading to a decline in its propelling and stimulating functions. The term is also known as the "occurrence of excess manifestations in extreme deficiency." For example, deficiency of spleen qi, causing dysfunction of transportation and transformation, may result in such pseudo-excess symptoms as gastric and abdominal distension and pain (usually intermittent). Another case in point is constipation that occurs after a prolonged or serious illness or in aged patients due to inability of deficient qi to propel bowel movement.

[**Previous Translation**] False sthenia-syndrome in appearance but real asthenia-syndrome in nature; REAL DEFICIENCY AND PSEUDO-EXCESS; sthenia-syndrome in appearance and asthenia-syndrome in nature; true deficiency with false excess; deficiency syndrome with pseudo-excess symptoms; real Deficiency with pseudo-Excess

[**Current Translation**] Deficiency syndrome with pseudo-excess symptoms; asthenia syndrome with pseudo-sthenia symptoms; true asthenia and false sthenia; true deficiency and false excess syndrome; true deficiency with false excess

[**Standard Translation**] True deficiency with pseudo-excess

Citations

- Moreover, average people are often found to have true deficiency pattern with pseudo-excess symptoms, and their eye diseases often fall into the pattern of upper heat and lower cold. (*The Great Compendium of Classics on Ophthalmology*)
- However, there may be excess manifestations when a deficiency pattern develops to an extreme, and thus pseudo-excess symptoms occur; there may be deficiency manifestations when an excess pattern develops to an extreme, and thus pseudo-deficiency symptoms occur. (*Medical Art*)

39. YĪNYÁNG SHĪTIÁO 阴阳失调

Yin-yang Disharmony

The term is a brief way to refer to the loss of balance between yin and yang. Specifically, it denotes that during the onset and development of a disease, the relative balance and coordination between yin and yang are broken due to various pathogenic factors, which results in a series of pathological changes including relative exuberance or debilitation, mutual impairment, mutual repelling, and collapse of yin and yang. The breakdown of balance between yin and yang primarily manifests itself as cold or heat patterns. In addition, traditional Chinese medicine believes that pathogenic qi will not cause illnesses until the yin-yang balance of the human body is broken. Therefore, in this sense, the term is also a general statement denoting various functional and organic disorders.

[Previous Translation] IMBALANCE OF YIN AND YANG; incoordination between yin and yang; yin-yang disharmony; imbalance of yin and yang; disharmony of yin and yang; imbalance of Yin and Yang; incoordination of Yin and Yang; imbalance/disorder of yin and yang

[Current Translation] Imbalance of yin and yang; imbalance between yin and yang; disharmony between yin and yang; yin-yang disharmony; breakdown of balance between yin and yang

[Standard Translation] Yin-yang disharmony

Citations

- All human diseases are caused by yin-yang disharmony or the relative predominance of water or fire. (*Feng's Secret Records in Brocade Bag*)
- All deficiency and impairment diseases are attributable to yin-yang disharmony or the relative predominance of water or fire. (*Comprehensive Secret Medical References of the Family*)

40. YĪNSHÈNG ZÉ HÁN 阴胜则寒

Yin Predominance Causes Cold

The term refers to the pathological state of excessive yin qi causing inhibition of physiological activities, excessive heat loss, and accumulation of pathogenic metabolites during disease development. While yin acts to cool, moisten, inhibit, and calm, pathogenic excess of yin featuring cold, inactivity, and dampness, with yang at a normal level, causes excess cold patterns. Clinically, it is manifested as cold body, cold limbs, lying curled up, pale and moist tongue, slow pulse, and so on. Yin predominance giving rise to cold manifestations is mainly attributable to yin pathogenic factors such as cold-dampness, overconsumption of raw or cold foods, and cold retained in the middle energizer, rendering yang qi in the body unable to counter excessive yin.

[Previous Translation] An excess of *yin* brings about cold-syndrome; PREDOMINANT YIN PRODUCES COLD; Excess of *yin* may lead to cold; excess of yin leading to cold syndromes; Cold syndromes of excess type will occur in cases of excess of yin; Predominance of yin leads to cold syndrome; Exuberant yin brings about endogenous cold; Excessive

Yin brings about Cold; excessive yin generating cold; hyper-yin generating cold

[**Current Translation**] Cold syndrome caused by an excess of yin; predominant yin leading to cold; predominance of yin leading to cold; abundance of yin producing cold manifestations; excessive yin giving rise to cold manifestations

[**Standard Translation**] Yin predominance causes cold.

Citations

- When malaria qi merges into yang aspect, yang has predominance; when it merges into yin aspect, yin has predominance. Yin predominance causes cold manifestations, while yang predominance causes heat manifestations. (*Plain Conversation*)
- In other words, chills and fever are the results of the struggle between yin and yang. Yin predominance causes cold manifestations, while yang predominance causes heat manifestations. (*Concise Exposition on Cold Damage*)
- Aversion to cold and fever is caused by the predominance of yin or yang. Yin predominance causes cold manifestations because of relative debilitation of yang; yang predominance causes heat manifestations because of relative debilitation of yin. (*Jingyue's Complete Works*)

41. YÁNGSHÈNG ZÉ RÈ 阳胜则热

Yang Predominance Causes Heat

The term refers to the pathological state of excessive yang qi causing hyperactivity, increased body responsiveness, and excessive heat during disease development. While yang acts to warm, propel, and excite, its pathological excess, characterized by heat, hyperactivity, and dryness, with yin at a normal level, results in excess heat pattern. Clinically, it is manifested as high fever, vexation, thirst, redness of face and eyes, dark yellow urine, dry stool, yellowish tongue coating, rapid pulse, and so on. Yang predominance giving rise to heat manifestations is mostly attributable to the attack by yang pathogenic factors such as warm-heat, the invasion by yin pathogenic factors which is transformed into heat, the damage from excessive emotions which turn into fire, and the heat resulting from depression due to qi stagnation, blood stasis, food accumulation, and so on.

[**Previous Translation**] An excess of *yang* may bring about heat-syndrome; excess of yang leading to heat syndromes; Heat syndromes of excess type will occur in cases of excess of yang; Exuberance of yang leads to heat syndrome; Excess of Yang brings about Heat syndrome; excessive yang generating heat; hyper-yang generating heat
[**Current Translation**] Heat syndrome due to an excess of yang; exuberance of yang generating heat; exuberant yang causing heat; heat syndrome brought about by extreme of yang; yang exuberance causing heat
[**Standard Translation**] Yang predominance causes heat.

Citations

- Aversion to cold and fever is caused by the predominance of yin or yang. Yin predominance causes cold manifestations because of relative debilitation of yang; yang predominance causes heat manifestations because of relative debilitation of yin. (*Jingyue's Complete Works*)
- Yin predominance causes cold manifestations, while yang predominance causes heat manifestations. The struggle between yin and yang leads to shivering and sweating at the same time. (*Annotated "Treatise on Cold Damage"*)
- According to *Yellow Emperor's Internal Canon of Medicine*, yang predominance may cause heat manifestations, which is the result of fire of excessive yang. Its clinical symptoms include vexation, thirst, dry stool, dark urine, difficult and painful urination, and surging rapid pulses on the six positions of the wrist. Herbal medicine cool or cold in property should be used for treatment. (*Stepping Stones for Medicine*)

42. YĪNSǓN JÍ YÁNG 阴损及阳

Yin Impairment Affects Yang

The term refers to the pathological state characterized by primary yin deficiency and secondary yang deficiency. Deficiency or impairment of yin essence or yin qi affects the generation of yang qi, or leads to the consumption of yang qi as yin and yang are mutually dependent, resulting in yang deficiency in addition to yin deficiency. For example, the pattern of liver-yang hyperactivity is caused mainly by deficiency of both liver yin and kidney yin, which fails to control yang, or, in terms of the five elements, water fails to nourish wood. However, the disease may progress to impair blood and essence of the liver and the kidney, which would affect the generation and transformation of kidney yang and bring symptoms of kidney-yang deficiency such as aversion to cold, cold limbs, brightly pale complexion, and deep thready pulse. Thus, deficiency of both yin and yang occurs as a result of yin impairment affecting yang.

[**Previous Translation**] Deficient *yin* affects *yang*; DEFICIENCY OF YIN AFFECTING YANG; *yang* involved by deficient *yin*; deficiency of yin affecting yang; impairment of yin affecting yang; Yin deficiency affects Yang; yin-consumption involving yang

[**Current Translation**] Deficiency of yin affecting yang; impairment of yin involving yang; detriment of yin affecting yang; yin impairment involving yang; impairment of yin impeding generation of yang; impairment of yin affecting yang; Detriment to yin affects yang; yin impairment affecting yang; syndrome/pattern of yin detriment affecting yang

[**Standard Translation**] Yin impairment affects yang.

Citations

- For cases caused by yin impairment affecting yang instead of six exogenous pathogenic factors, therapies of dredging and/or purgation could be used and stomach yin should be nourished. (*Case Records: A Guide to Clinical Practice*)
- The patient recently felt cold, and did not feel hungry with no desire to eat. This is a case of yin impairment affecting yang. (*Case Records of Elderly Yipiao in Saoye House*)

43. YÁNGSŬN JÍ YĪN 阳损及阴

Yang Impairment Affects Yin

The term refers to the pathological state characterized by primary yang deficiency and secondary yin deficiency. Deficiency or impairment of yang qi affects the generation of yin qi as yin and yang are mutually dependent, resulting in yin deficiency in addition to yang deficiency. For example, edema is caused mainly by deficiency of kidney yang. Deficient kidney yang fails to transform qi, which leads to disturbance of water metabolism and hence retention of body fluids in the skin. However, the disease may progress to deficiency of yin qi as deficient yang qi fails to generate sufficient yin qi and manifests symptoms of kidney-yin deficiency such as worsening emaciation and even convulsion as a result of stirring of wind due to ascending yang. Thus, deficiency of both yin and yang occurs as a result of yang impairment affecting yin.

[**Previous Translation**] Deficient *yang* affects *yin*; DEFICIENCY OF YANG AFFECTING YIN; *yin* involved by the deficient *yang*; weakness of yang affecting yin; impairment of yang affecting yin; Yang damages Yin; Deficiency of Yang affects Yin; yang consumption involving yin

[**Current Translation**] Deficiency of yang affecting yin; impairment of yang affecting yin; impairment of yang involving yin; yang impairment involving yin; impairment of yang impeding generation of yin; detriment to yang affects yin; yang impairment affecting yin; syndrome/ pattern of yang detriment affecting yin

[**Standard Translation**] Yang impairment affects yin.

Citations

- Heart failure is caused by yin impairment affecting yang and yang impairment affecting yin, resulting in impairment of both yin and yang, accompanied with excessive retained morbid fluids and phlegm. (*100 Contemporary TCM Clinicians Series: Shi Zhichao*)
- Kidney yang impairment affects yin and may lead to deficiency of both yin and yang, and even manifest as consumptive disease. (*Pattern Differentiation Based on Pathogenesis in Traditional Chinese Medicine*)

44. YÁNGSHÈNG ZÉ YĪNBÌNG 阳胜则阴病

Yang Predominance Causes Yin Disorder

The term refers to various pathological changes characterized by impairment of body fluids and yin due to predominance of yang heat. As yang becomes exuberant and its damage to yin is not yet obvious, excess heat pattern will occur. If the condition worsens, that is, yang heat becomes increasingly excessive and causes obvious damage to yin in the body, the disease will progress from excess heat pattern to the pattern of excess heat accompanied with yin deficiency. In the long run, as yin might be damaged to a great extent, the disease may further develop from excess heat pattern into deficiency-heat pattern.

[**Previous Translation**] An excess of *yang* leads to weakness of *yin*; EXCESS OF YANG CAUSING DISORDER OF YIN; An excess of *yang* leads to deficiency of *yin*; Predominance of Yang Consumes Yin; predominance of yang leading to disorder of yin; yang excess causing yin deficiency; hyper-yang causing hypo-yin

[**Current Translation**] Disorder of yin caused by an excess of yang; exuberance of yang leading to disorder of yin; exuberant yang leading to disorder of yin; yang in excess making yin suffer; predominant yang making yin disorder; predominance of yang leading to disorder of yin

[**Standard Translation**] Yang predominance causes yin disorder.

Citations

- Yin predominance causes yang disorder, giving rise to cold manifestations, while yang predominance causes yin disorder, giving rise to heat manifestations. (*Plain Conversation*)
- Yin predominance leads to yang deficiency, and yang predominance leads to yin deficiency. In other words, yin predominance causes yang disorder and yang predominance causes yin disorder. (*Formulas for Pattern Treatment to Safeguard Life, Part II*)

45. YĪNSHÈNG ZÉ YÁNGBÌNG 阴胜则阳病

Yin Predominance Causes Yang Disorder

The term refers to the pathological change of yang-qi decline caused by predominance of yin cold. Excessive yin cold in the body will impair yang qi in the long run, causing yang deficiency characterized by a decrease in physiological functions of the body and insufficiency of yang heat. Thus, symptoms of both excess cold and yang deficiency manifest themselves. If yin predominance has damaged yang for a long time, yang qi will be seriously impaired, and the disease may progress from an excess pattern to a deficiency-cold pattern.

[**Previous Translation**] An excess of *yin* leads to weakness of *yang*; EXCESS OF YIN CAUSING DISORDER OF YANG; An excess of *yin* leads to deficiency of *yang*; Predominance of Yin Consumes Yang; Predominant yin leads to disorder of yang; Excess of Yin leads to disorder of Yang; yin excess causing yang deficiency; hyper-yin causing hypo-yang

[**Current Translation**] Disorder of yang due to an excess of yin; predominant yin leading to yang disease; yin in excess making yang suffer; excessive yin making yang suffer; predominant yin making yang disorder; predominance of yin leading to disorder of yang

[**Standard Translation**] Yin predominance causes yang disorder.

Citations

- Deficiency of yang qi will make yin relatively excessive, and cold signs and symptoms may occur. Therefore, yin predominance causes yang disorder and cold manifestations occur. (*Jingyue's Complete Works*)
- Pathological changes of yin will lead to blood stasis, which causes predominance of yin. Yin predominance may cause yang disorder. (*Original Decrees of Medicine*)

46. YĪNSHÈNG GÉYÁNG 阴盛格阳

Exuberant Yin Repels Yang

The term, also known as repelling yang, refers to the pathological state in which extremely exuberant yin cold is congested inside the body, forcing yang qi to flow to the body surface. Excessive internal yin cold is the fundamental cause of the disease. However, as yang qi is repelled by yin cold and driven to the body surface, pseudo-heat symptoms may appear such as red face, vexing heat, thirst, and apparently surging pulse without root in addition to the original symptoms of excessive yin in the interior such as pale complexion, reversal cold of the limbs, listlessness, and feeble pulse. Thus, it is described as the pattern of true cold with pseudo-heat. Clinically, a disease known as "floating yang" is also a manifestation of exuberant yin repelling yang. It is characterized by lower cold in nature and upper heat in disguise as a result of the failure of yin and yang to maintain each other when true yang (kidney qi) is extremely weak and fails to restrict yin and yin becomes excessive in the body and drives the feeble yang to the upper part of the body.

[**Previous Translation**] *Yang* is kept externally by the excessive *yin* inside the body; EXCESSIVE YIN HINDERS YANG; excessive *yin* repelling yang; exuberant yin repelling yang; Excessive Yin keeps Yang externally; excessive yin rejecting yang

[**Current Translation**] Yang kept externally by yin excess in the interior; predominant yin rejecting yang; exuberant yin repelling yang; excessive yin repelling yang; pseudo-heat manifestations in the exterior due to extreme cold in the interior; syndrome/pattern of exuberant yin with repelled yang

[**Standard Translation**] Exuberant yin repels yang.

Citations

- Patients who suffer from cold damage with exuberant yin repelling yang are found to have cold sensation, thready deep rapid or racing pulse, vexation, and no desire to drink water. (*Brief Cases of Yin Pattern*)
- In the cases of pseudo-heat pattern, water becomes extremely excessive, like fire, making yin pattern appear like yang pattern…. It is also described as exuberant yin repelling yang. (*Orthodoxy of Medicine*)
- If a patient has had cold damage for less than three days and feels cold with sweat on the forehead, redness of face, and vexation, it is not a case of yin-toxin pattern, but exuberant yin repelling yang. (*Symptoms, Causes, Pulses, and Treatments*)

47. YÁNgSHÈNg gÉYĪN 阳盛格阴

Exuberant Yang Repels Yin

The term, also known as repelling yin, refers to the pathological state in which extremely exuberant yang heat is hidden deeply inside the body, or in other words, yang qi is obstructed inside the body and fails to flow to the body surface while yin qi is driven out. Exuberant yang in the interior is the fundamental cause of the disease. However, as yin qi is repelled by yang heat and driven to the body surface, symptoms of pseudo-cold such as reversal cold of the limbs as well as deep hidden pulse may appear in addition to the original symptoms of excessive internal heat pathogen in the interior such as high fever, redness of face, heavy breathing, vexation, red tongue, and forceful rapid surging pulse. Thus, it is called the pattern of true heat with pseudo-cold.

[**Previous Translation**] *Yin* is kept externally by the excessive *yang* inside the body; EXCESSIVE YANG HINDERS YIN; *yin* is kept superficially by excessive *yang* inside body; Exuberant yang repels yin; Excessive Yang keeps Yin externally; excessive yang rejecting yin
[**Current Translation**] Yin kept externally by yang excess in the interior; exuberant yang repelling yin; superabundant yang rejecting yin; pseudo-cold manifestations in the exterior due to extreme heat in the interior
[**Standard Translation**] Exuberant yang repels yin.

Citations

- In the cases of pseudo-cold pattern, fire becomes extremely excessive, like water, making yang pattern appear like yin pattern.... It is also described as exuberant yang repelling yin. (*Orthodoxy of Medicine*)
- Exuberant yang repelling yin causes a pattern like that of yin, manifested as cold pain in the body surface, cold limbs, but forceful deep rapid pulse. It is an indication for *Chengqi* Decoction (Purgative Decoction). (*Symptoms, Causes, Pulses, and Treatments*)
- In the cases of febrile diseases, if aversion to cold occurs but with dry mouth and throat, yellowish tongue, and chapped lips, it is the manifestation of exuberant yang repelling yin, that is, there is excess heat in the interior with cold signs and symptoms in the exterior. It is not truly aversion to cold. (*Systematic Differentiation of Cold Damage and Warm Epidemics*)

48. YÁNgwēi YĪNXIÁN 阳微阴弦

Faint Pulse at Yang and Wiry Pulse at Yin

The term refers to faint pulse at the *cun* (寸) section and wiry pulse at the *chi* (尺) section, the pulse manifestations of chest impediment and heart pain from the perspective of pathogenesis. Pulse at the *cun* section is yang, while pulse at the *chi* section is yin. The faint pulse at the *cun* section indicates insufficiency of yang qi in the upper energizer and hypofunction of yang qi in the chest. The wiry pulse at the *chi* section shows yin-cold excess and water retention. The concurrence of two pulse manifestations indicates that chest impediment and heart pain are caused by yang deficiency in the upper energizer leading to the attack of the upper energizer by yin pathogens and fight between pathogenic qi and healthy qi. According to the section "Pulses, Patterns, and Treatments of Diseases of Chest Impediment, Heart Pain, and Shortness of Breath" in *Essential Prescriptions of the Golden Cabinet*, "Now through examination, it is known that yang deficiency exists in the upper energizer. The chest impediment and heart pain are attributable to the fight between yin and yang as is indicated by wiry pulse at yin (the *chi* section)." This further illustrates that the manifestations of faint pulse at yang and wiry pulse at yin are indispensable aspects of the etiology and pathogenesis of chest impediment and heart pain.

[**Previous Translation**] /
[**Current Translation**] Weak pulse at yang and wiry pulse at yin
[**Standard Translation**] Faint pulse at yang and wiry pulse at yin

Citations

- Pay attention to excess and insufficiency when taking pulse. Faint pulse at yang (the *cun* section) and wiry pulse at yin (the *chi* section) indicate chest impediment and heart pain. The underlying cause is that yang qi is extremely weak. (*Essential Prescriptions of the Golden Cabinet*)
- The pulse manifestation of chest impediment is faint pulse at yang and wiry pulse at yin. Faint pulse at yang means the disease is in the upper energizer, and wiry pulse at yin means heart pain may appear. Hence, the therapy of unblocking yang should be adopted according to *Essential Prescriptions of the Golden Cabinet* and *Important Formulas Worth a Thousand Gold Pieces*. (*Categorized Patterns with Clear-Cut Treatments*)
- Deep slow radial pulse as well as faint pulse at yang and wiry pulse at yin indicates that it is a case of cold pattern, not heat pattern. (*Case Records: A Guide to Clinical Practice*)

49. QÌJĪ SHĪTIÁO 气机失调

Qi Movement Disorder

The term refers to the pathological changes of inhibited qi flow or uncoordinated and imbalanced ascending, descending, exiting, and entering of qi. According to traditional Chinese medicine, normal movement of qi should be smooth, unimpeded, coordinated, and balanced; otherwise, it is known as qi movement disorder. Due to the diversity of qi movement, there are various manifestations of qi movement disorder. For example, qi stagnation means the movement of qi is obstructed, constrained, inhibited, and stagnated, resulting in distention, oppression, and pain. Qi counterflow refers to excessive ascending or insufficient descending of qi, mostly causing pathological changes of the lung, the stomach, the liver, and other zang-fu organs. Qi sinking refers to inadequate ascending or excessive descending of qi, marked by sinking of qi as qi is deficient and unable to lift. Qi block means that qi movement is constrained and blocked, and qi fails to exit, leading to the obstruction of clear orifices, featured by fainting and unconsciousness. Qi collapse means that qi fails to stay inside the body and flows outside in large amounts, resulting in a sudden complete failure of body functions.

[**Previous Translation**] /
[**Current Translation**] Disorder of qi movement; qi movement disorder
[**Standard Translation**] Qi movement disorder

Citations

- *Renshen* Powder (Ginseng Powder) is used to treat five kinds of dysphagia, namely, qi stagnation in gastric cavity, fullness and oppression in the heart and chest, obstruction in the throat, disorder of qi movement, and inability to eat. (*Formulas for Universal Relief*)
- As filth and dampness remain inside the body, yellowish tongue coating, gastric distension and fullness, as well as qi movement disorder occur. Over time, heat is generated. The Third Variant *Zheng Qi* Powder (Qi-correcting Powder) should be used. (*Systematic Differentiation of Warm Diseases*)

50. YÍNGWÈI BÙHÉ 营卫不和

Nutrient-Defense Disharmony

The term refers to the disharmony between nutrient qi and defense qi. Nutrient qi or nutrient corresponds to yin and stays in the interior, and defense qi or defense corresponds to yang and defends in the exterior. In physiological state, defense qi, which flows outside the vessels, protects fleshy exterior and warms as well as nourishes muscles, skin, and body hair. It also regulates and controls the opening and closing of striae and interstices as well as the excretion of sweat, and so on. Nutrient qi, which flows inside the vessels, nourishes and moistens the zang-fu organs, limbs, and skeleton. Harmony and coordination between nutrient qi and defense qi are an important prerequisite for normal functioning of human body and defense of health against external pathogens. If the body is weak, or externally contracts wind pathogen, disharmony between nutrient qi and defense qi will occur. As a result, yang qi fails to secure the exterior and yin fluids tend to be excreted easily, resulting in symptoms such as fever, spontaneous sweating, and fear of cold or wind. Nutrient-defense disharmony can be found in cases of external contraction of wind pathogen or miscellaneous internal diseases.

[**Previous Translation**] Imbalance between *ying*-energy and *wei*-energy; DISHARMONY BETWEEN YING (NUTRIENTS) AND WEI (DEFENSE MECHANISM); derangement between nutrient and defensive qi; disharmony between nutrient qi and defensive qi; disharmony between nutrient Qi and defensive Qi

[**Current Translation**] Disharmony between nutritive-qi and defensive-qi; disharmony between ying qi and wei qi; disharmony between nutrient qi and defensive qi; disharmony between nutrient and defense; disharmony between ying and wei systems; disharmony between nutrient and defense (systems); nutrient-defense disharmony; disharmony between nutrient and defensive qi; syndrome/pattern of nutrient qi and defense qi disharmony

[**Standard Translation**] Nutrient-defense disharmony

Citations

- Even if such symptoms of nutrient-defense disharmony as floating pulse and spontaneous sweating do not fall into the cases of externally contracted disease, they are indications for *Guizhi* Decoction (Cinnamon Twig Decoction). (*Continued Treatise on Cold Damage*)
- In cases of nutrient-defense disharmony, vessels must have been obstructed, so *shaoyao* (*Radix Paeoniae Alba seu Rubra*, white or red peony root), *gancao* (*Radix et Rhizoma Glycyrrhizae*, licorice root), and *dazao* (*Fructus Jujubae*, Chinese date) should be used to harmonize nutrient and defense aspects. (*Effective Use of Established Formulas*)
- The stagnation of qi and blood, together with nutrient-defense disharmony, leads to irregular periods in timing and/or quantity. (*Remnants of Medical Decree*)

51. YÍNGRUÒ WÈIQIÁNG 营弱卫强

Weak Nutrient and Strong Defense

The term refers to the pathogenesis of *taiyang* (greater yang) wind-invasion pattern, that is, defense yang floats outside and nutrient yin fails to stay inside the body. Wind is a yang pathogen and attacks the defense exterior. When pathogenic wind invades, defense qi, which ascends, dissipates, and moves, floats out to body surface to fight against the wind pathogen, resulting in fever. Being opening and dispersing, the pathogenic wind makes the defense exterior become insecure and fail to keep nutrient qi in the interior, resulting in spontaneous sweating. As interstitial space enlarges and muscles relax with perspiration, human body cannot defend against the wind pathogen, and aversion to wind may occur. Due to the weakness of nutrient qi and the dispersing nature of wind, the pulse of the patient is floating and moderate. In sum, the main symptoms of *taiyang* wind-invasion pattern include fever, aversion to wind, spontaneous sweating, and floating moderate pulse.

[Previous Translation] /
[Current Translation] Weakness of nutritive-qi and hyper-activities of the defensive qi; strong defense with weak nutrient (卫强营弱); excess of defense qi and deficiency of nutrient qi (卫强营弱)
[Standard Translation] Weak nutrient and strong defense

Citations

- *Taiyang* disease characterized by fever and perspiration indicates weak nutrient and strong defense. That is why there is perspiration. The appropriate formula for treating diseases caused by wind pathogen is *Guizhi* Decoction (Cinnamon Twig Decoction). (*Treatise on Cold Damage*)
- This is to explain the quotation of "floating defense yang resulting in fever and weak nutrient yin resulting in perspiration" in the previous article. It means such symptoms are caused by weak nutrient and strong defense. Nutrient qi becomes weaker due to the loss of body fluids, while defense qi becomes stronger due to the invasion of pathogenic wind. (*Medical Warnings*)

52. YÍNGQIÁNG WÈIRUÒ 营强卫弱

Strong Nutrient and Weak Defense

The term refers to the pathogens is of *taiyang* cold-damage pattern, that is, nutrient yin is constrained and defense yang obstructed. Cold is a yin pathogen and is prone to attack nutrient yin. When pathogenic cold invades, nutrient qi, due to its increase in descent and inactivity, obstructs the defense qi in the interior, making defense qi unable to disperse on body surface to warm the skin, and thus aversion to cold occurs. When yang qi is obstructed inside and unable to disperse, fever also occurs. Moreover, when pathogenic cold fetters the exterior and blocks the pores, absence of sweating and floating tight pulse could be found. Finally, defense-nutrient disharmony and obstructed meridians and collaterals could result in headache, painful stiff nape, and painful joints. In sum, the main symptoms of *taiyang* exterior excess pattern include fever, aversion to cold, absence of sweating, headache, painful stiff nape, painful joints, and floating tight pulse.

[Previous Translation] /
[Current Translation] Weak defense with strong nutrient (卫弱营强); weak defense qi and strong nutrient (卫弱营强); deficiency of defense qi and excess of nutrient qi (卫弱营强)
[Standard Translation] Strong nutrient and weak defense

Citations

- As pathogenic cold invades nutrient aspect, excess pattern of nutrient aspect and deficiency pattern of defense aspect would be found. The symptoms include absence of sweating and aversion to wind as a result of strong nutrient (due to stagnation) and weak defense (due to being constrained). (*Profound Significance and Ingenious Uses of the "Treatise on Cold Damage"*)
- *Mahuang* Decoction (Ephedra Decoction) which induces sweating should be used to relieve panting caused by ascending counterflow of qi due to strong nutrient and weak defense. (*Direct Guidance on Cold Damage*)

53. WŬZHÌ HUÀ HUŎ 五志化火

Five Emotions Transform into Fire

The term refers to the pathological change caused by excess of five emotions and mental activities, namely, anger, joy, over-thinking, sorrow, and fear. In the long run, they generate heat and transform into fire. "Five emotions transforming into fire" or "the excess of five emotions transforming into fire" refers to the pathological changes caused by mental and emotional overstimulation, which affects coordination and balance of the zang-fu organs, essential qi, and yin and yang, leading to yang excess, hyperactivity, and counterflow in zang-fu organs, or causes constraint and stagnation of qi, transforming into yang and fire if such qi constraint and stagnation lasts for a long time. For instance, internal damage caused by uncontrolled emotions and depression often leads to liver qi constraint and stagnation, which then transforms into liver fire. Another example is that anger damages the liver, leading to hyperactivity and counterflow of liver qi, which may transform into liver fire.

[**Previous Translation**] Fire-syndrome caused by the disorders of the five emotions; FIVE EMOTIONS PRODUCING FIRE; fire syndrome caused by the disorders of five emotions; five emotions transforming into fire; Five excessive emotions convert into internal Fire

[**Current Translation**] Heat syndromes caused by the disorders of five emotions; five emotions transforming into fire; fire syndrome triggered by emotional stress; transformation of five emotions into fire; transformation of the five minds into fire; five minds transforming into fire [**Standard Translation**] Five emotions transform into fire.

Citations

- Liu Hejian once said that excessive five emotions can transform into fire. (*Danxi's Mastery of Medicine*)
- Vexation and overstrain may lead to excessive five emotions, which may transform into fire and result in stroke. The pathogenesis is that extreme heat produces fire. (*Case Records: A Guide to Clinical Practice*)
- In addition, some patients suffer from stroke because of excessive five emotions which can transform into intense internal heat. Those who believe that such stroke is caused by wind only see the branch and forget the root. (*Comprehensive Medicine by Doctor Zhang Lu*)

54. GĀNYÁNG HUÀ FĒNG 肝阳化风

Liver Yang Transforms into Wind

The term refers to the pathological change due to depletion of liver yin and kidney yin, in which the kidney (water) fails to nourish the liver (wood), and thus, hyperactivity and counterflow of liver yang without restriction stir wind. In most cases, liver yang transforming into wind is due to the constraint of emotions which causes internal damage and transforms into fire, and hence damages yin. Another possibility is that overstrain consumes and damages liver yin and kidney yin, causing yin deficiency and yang hyperactivity. Thus, liver yang floats and cannot be subdued, whose hyperactivity and counterflow transform into stirring wind. Clinically, it is manifested as dizziness, proneness to forward fall, muscle twitching, limb numbness and tremor, facial palsy, or hemiplegia. In severe cases, sudden forward fall may occur due to the counterflow of qi and blood such as wind-stroke block and wind-stroke collapse. Liver yang transforming into wind is often seen in the cases of wind-stroke.

[**Previous Translation**] Liver-Yang changes into Liver-Wind
[**Current Translation**] Interior wind caused by excessive liver-yang; liver-yang transforming into wind; transformation of liver yang into fire; syndrome/pattern of liver yang transforming into wind
[**Standard Translation**] Liver yang transforms into wind.

Citations

- Ascending counterflow of qi from the liver carries ministerial fire with it, so most qi-related diseases manifest the pathogenesis of counterflow of liver qi invading the stomach or hyperactive liver yang transforming into wind. (*Categorized Patterns with Clear-cut Treatments*)
- Racing pulse at the left hand of the patient and soggy pulse at the right hand indicate kidney-yin deficiency, which fails to nourish and moisten the liver, and thus, liver yang becomes hyperactive and transforms into wind. (*Case Records: A Guide to Clinical Practice*)
- Hyperactive liver yang transforms into wind, its transverse invasion affecting the spleen and the stomach, leading to transportation and transformation disorder. As a result, water-dampness that has not been transported away accumulates to form phlegm, which flows in the collaterals of the liver and the gallbladder. (*Case Records of Jingxiang Mansion*)

55. YĪNXŪ SHĒNg FĒNG 阴虚生风

Yin Deficiency Generates Wind

The term refers to the pathological change due to the exhaustion of liver yin and kidney yin giving rise to sinews being deprived of nourishment and wind being stirred internally. Yin deficiency generating wind is often caused by yin-fluid insufficiency in the late stage of febrile diseases, yin consumption due to chronic diseases, or natural consumption of yin fluids in the liver and the kidney due to aging. Insufficiency makes yin fluids unable to nourish and moisten sinews and vessels, which produces internal wind. Clinically, it is manifested as limb wriggling and muscle twitching, accompanied with such symptoms of yin exhaustion as tidal low-grade fever, night sweat, bone steaming, red tongue with little coating and saliva, and thready rapid weak pulse. As this is a pathological change of deficiency in nature, its symptoms of stirring wind are mostly mild and moderate and commonly seen in elderly patients and patients with sequelae of externally contracted febrile diseases or chronic illnesses.

[Previous Translation] /
[Current Translation] Interior wind due to yin deficiency; yin-asthenia producing wind; yin deficiency generating wind
[Standard Translation] Yin deficiency generates wind.

Citations

- It denotes yin deficiency generates wind rather than external contraction of pathogenic qi. (*Delving into the Description of Materia Medica*)
- Qi deficiency generates phlegm, and yin deficiency generates wind. Wind pathogen with phlegm runs through the meridians, resulting in stiff joints. (*Case Records of Chen Lianfang*)
- Cases of liver-and-stomach yin deficiency, in which wind is generated and limb atrophy occurs, could be treated with dredging and astringing therapies. Medicinal substances to be used include *shudi* (Radix Rehmanniae Praeparata, prepared rehmannia root), *niuxi* (Radix Achyranthis Bidentatae, two-toothed achyranthes root), *yuanzhi* (Radix Polygalae, thin-leaf milkwort root), *qizi* (Fructus Lycii, Chinese wolfberry fruit), *shihu* (Caulis Dendrobii, dendrobium stem), and *gouteng* (Ramulus Uncariae Cum Uncis, gambir plant). (*Categorized Patterns with Clear-Cut Treatments*)

56. XUÈXŪ SHĒNG FĒNG 血虚生风

Blood Deficiency Generates Wind

The term refers to the pathological change due to blood deficiency giving rise to poor nourishment of sinews and internal stirring of deficient wind. It is often caused by insufficient blood production or massive blood loss. Another cause is insufficient liver blood failing to nourish the sinews due to the consumption and damage of nutrient blood caused by chronic diseases. The third reason is that blood fails to nourish collaterals. Clinically, it is manifested as limb numbness, sinew and muscle twitching, and even limb tremor and spasms, accompanied by symptoms of blood deficiency. As this pathological change is a deficiency pattern in nature, its symptoms of stirring wind are relatively mild and moderate.

[**Previous Translation**] Deficiency of blood may cause wind syndrome; blood deficiency producing wind; Wind syndrome due to Blood Deficiency

[**Current Translation**] Interior wind due to blood deficiency; blood-asthenia generating wind; blood deficiency producing wind; blood deficiency producing wind; generation of endogenous wind due to blood deficiency; syndrome/pattern of blood deficiency with generation of wind; pattern/syndrome of blood deficiency engendering wind; blood deficiency producing wind; syndrome/pattern of blood deficiency producing wind

[**Standard Translation**] Blood deficiency generates wind.

Citations

- If convulsive seizure or similar symptoms occur, it is because blood deficiency in the liver meridian generates wind. *Siwu* Decoction (Four Ingredients Decoction) plus *tianma* (*Rhizoma Gastrodiae*, tall gastrodis tuber) and *goutenggou* (*Ramulus Uncariae Cum Uncis*, gambir plant) should be used for treatment. (*Comprehensive Medicine by Doctor Zhang Lu*)
- For patients with massive blood loss and whose blood deficiency generates wind, *Xiaoyao* Powder (Free Wanderer Powder) should be used with *chuanxiong* (*Rhizoma Chuanxiong*, Sichuan lovage rhizome), *qingxiangzi* (*Semen Celosiae*, feather cockscomb seed), and *xiakucao* (*Spica Prunellae*, common self-heal fruit-spike). (*Treatise on Blood Syndromes*)
- *Duhuo Jisheng* Decoction (Pubescent Angelica and Mistletoe Decoction) is mainly used to treat postpartum symptoms of blood deficiency generating wind such as convulsion of hands and feet, sinew spasms and tension, frequent muscle twitching, and hemiplegia. (*Effective Formulas from Generations of Physicians*)

57. RÈJÍ SHĒNG FĒNG 热极生风

Extreme Heat Generates Wind

The term refers to the pathological change caused by intense pathogenic heat which damages nutrient blood, scorches the liver meridian, and deprives sinews of nourishment, leading to spasm, tension, and convulsion. Its pathogenesis is that intense pathogenic heat dries body fluids, damages nutrient blood, scorches the liver meridian, and causes sinews to become stiff and taut. Clinically, it is manifested as convulsive syncope, convulsion of the limbs, showing the whites of eyes, and opisthotonos, accompanied with high fever, loss of consciousness, delirious speech, and so on. As its pathogenesis is attributable to the hyperactivity of heat pathogen, it is an excess pattern in nature, often seen at the fastigium of externally contracted febrile diseases.

[**Previous Translation**] EXTREME HEAT BRINGING ABOUT WIND; extreme heat causing wind; Extreme Heat causes Wind; overheat generating wind
[**Current Translation**] Interior wind due to overabundance of pathogenic heat; extreme heat producing wind; excessive heat generating wind; extreme heat producing wind; intense heat generating wind; syndrome/pattern of extreme heat with generation of wind; extreme heat engendering wind; extreme heat producing wind
[**Standard Translation**] Extreme heat generates wind.

Citations

- Or extreme heat generates wind, i.e., internal constraint of dryness-heat causes stiff tongue, lockjaw, and muscle twitching. (*Profound Formulas Inspired by the Yellow Emperor's Plain Conversation*)
- Most pediatric diseases are caused by extreme heat generating wind, which leads to infantile convulsion, so heat should be cleared as soon as it appears. (*Concise Medical Guidelines*)
- This therapy is used to treat the pattern of extreme heat generating wind, so *lianqiao* (*Fructus Forsythiae*, weeping forsythia capsule) and *zhuye* (*Folium Phyllostachydis Henonis*, henon bamboo leaf) are used to clear the heat. (*Treatise on Seasonal Diseases*)

58. XUÈZÀO SHĒNG FĒNG 血燥生风

Blood Dryness Generates Wind

The term refers to the pathological change manifested as dry and itchy skin as well as desquamation caused by the deficiency of blood and fluids which fail to moisten and nourish the muscles and skin. Blood dryness generating endogenous wind is often caused by consumption of essence and blood due to chronic diseases, deficiency of essence and blood due to senility, insufficiency of blood generation due to long-term improper diet, or malfunction of blood generation due to accumulation of static blood, leading to depletion of fluids and blood which brings failure to moisten and nourish the muscles and skin and transforming into wind. Clinically, it is marked by dry or scaly skin, itching, and skin desquamation.

[Previous Translation] Blood-dryness producing endogenous wind
[Current Translation] Blood dryness generating/producing wind; Dryness in blood generates internal wind; blood dryness causing wind; blood dryness producing wind
[Standard Translation] Blood-dryness generates wind.

Citations

- Urticaria in women is caused by the anger-fire in the liver meridian and the endogenous wind due to blood dryness. (*Complete Effective Prescriptions for Women's Diseases*)
- Dry skin, thinness, itching, pain, bleeding from scratches, or white scurf, without bleeding, from scratches are caused by endogenous wind due to blood dryness and the heat resulting from constrained wind. (*Collection of Case Records in External Patterns*)
- Patients with blood dryness generating wind in the liver meridian should be treated with nourishing kidney water and engendering liver blood, which quenches the fire and extinguishes the wind to stop itching. (*Jingyue's Complete Works*)

59. TŬYŌNG MÙYÙ 土壅木郁

Earth Stagnation and Wood Depression

The term refers to the pathological change in which the stagnation of spleen qi and its disorder of ascending and descending cause the failure of the liver to govern the free flow of qi. It is also known as liver depression due to spleen dampness, or earth counter-restricting wood as the spleen pertains to earth and the liver pertains to wood according to the five-element theory. Improper diet impairs the spleen and the stomach, causing the failure of the spleen to transport and the occurrence of internal dampness. The spleen earth is thus encumbered, incurring qi stagnation in the middle energizer and its disorder of ascending and descending, making the liver unbale to govern the free flow of qi. Clinically, it is marked by poor digestion, abdominal distention, poor appetite, loose stools, and greasy tongue coating due to dampness encumbering the spleen. Subsequent symptoms include hypochondriac pain and mental depression caused by liver-qi stagnation. Bitter taste in mouth and jaundice may occur if damp-heat encumbers the spleen to affect the liver in governing the free flow of qi, causing the counterflow and overflow of bile.

[Previous Translation] /
[Current Translation] Earth stagnation and wood depression
[Standard Translation] Earth stagnation and wood depression

Citations

- Patients with stomach disorders present symptoms such as abdominal distension, and pain in the upper stomach near the precordium, with obstructive feeling in the hypochondriac region where the liver meridian travels. They are manifestations of spleen-qi stagnation causing the failure of the liver to govern the free flow of qi. (*Classified Compilation and Concise Annotation of "Plain Conversation" and "Spiritual Pivot"*)
- The spleen governs muscles, and thus excess of the body indicates spleen dampness encumbers the liver and the liver fails to govern the free flow of qi, presenting with symptoms of abdominal distension and inhibited urination and defecation. (*Explanation of Unresolved Issues in "Plain Conversation"*)

- Binding of phlegm and qi causes stagnation of spleen qi and depression of liver qi, giving rise to liver dysfunction. (*Case Records of Zhang Yuqing*)

60. TǓ BÙ ZHÌSHUǏ 土不制水

Earth Fails to Control Water

The term refers to the pathological change characterized by stagnation and overflow of damp-turbidity due to weak spleen earth failing to transport, transform, and control fluids and dampness. According to the five-element theory, the spleen pertains to earth and the kidney pertains to water. Normally spleen earth controls water to achieve proper transportation and transformation, preventing pathological overflow. However, when spleen earth is weak and fails to control water, overflow problems may occur and symptoms such as edema and phlegm-rheum can be found.

[**Previous Translation**] INHIBITION OF EARTH TO TRANSPORT WATER; Earth fails to control water; Earth fails to restrain water; Spleen fails to restrict Water (Kidney)
[**Current Translation**] Earth fails to restrict water; earth failing to control water; failure of earth to restrain water; spleen failing to restrain kidney; earth (spleen) failing to control water (kidney)
[**Standard Translation**] Earth fails to control water.

Citations

- Deficient kidney yang is unable to warm spleen yang, causing the weakness of spleen earth and its failure to control water. Thus, there may occur frenetic flowing of water, obstruction in the waterway of triple energizer, and blocking of qi in meridians. When qi movement in the human body is impaired, panting consequently occurs; when uncontrolled water permeates the meridians and collaterals, edema occurs, especially in the legs, feet, and under the eyes. (*Discussion of Pathology Based on Triple Etiology Doctrine*)
- Usually with declined spleen qi and exhausted original qi, spleen earth is too weak to control water so that water overflow problems occur. (*Reserved Formulas of Yang's Family*)

- Phlegm is transformed from water, originating from the kidney and produced by the spleen... That phlegm is produced by the spleen is due to the failure of the spleen to transport and transform food and drinks as well as to control water and dampness. (*Jingyue's Complete Works*)

61. MÙHUǑ XÍNG JĪN 木火刑金

Wood Fire Impairs Metal

The term refers to the pathological change caused by the ascending counterflow of intense liver fire impairing the lung to purify qi. It is also known as liver fire invading the lung. According to the five-element theory, the liver pertains to wood and the lung pertains to metal, hence the name. Physiologically, liver qi ascends, while lung qi descends. They are opposite but complementary, restricting each other to prevent excess or insufficiency. If liver qi is constrained, qi depression can transform into fire, and fire may scorch the lung collaterals and impair the lung to purify qi. Hence, clinical symptoms may occur including vexation, irritability, chest and hypochondriac pain, bitter taste in mouth, redness of eyes, cough, dyspnea, and hemoptysis.

[**Previous Translation**] WOOD FIRE DAMAGING METAL; Wood-fire impairs metal; Wood-Fire Burns Metal
[**Current Translation**] Wood-fire impairing metal; wood fire tormenting metal; wood (liver) fire tormenting metal (lung)
[**Standard Translation**] Wood fire impairs metal.

Citations

- Cough with blood, loss of voice, emaciation, and redness of face are the symptoms of wood fire impairing metal and should be treated accordingly. (*Case Records of Elderly Yipiao in Saoye House*)
- Cough due to wood fire impairing metal should be treated with *Zhisou* Powder (Cough-stopping Powder) plus *chaihu* (*Radix Bupleuri*, Chinese thorowax root), *zhiqiao* (*Fructus Aurantii*, orange fruit), and *chishao* (*Radix Paeoniae Rubra*, peony root). (*Bihua's Medical Works*)

- Persistent coughing and chocking, even vomiting and nausea, caused by wood fire impairing metal should be treated mainly by clearing the liver and moistening the lung. (*Case Records of Ganshan Cottage*)

62. ZǏ DÀO MǓQÌ 子盗母气

Child Organ Affects Mother Organ

The term refers to the pathogenesis of deficient child organ affecting mother organ in accordance with the generation among the five elements (i.e., zang-organs). For instance, spleen earth is the mother organ and lung metal is the child organ. The deficiency of lung qi can affect the spleen, that is, child organ affects mother organ, thus impairing the transportation of spleen qi and causing the lack of source in transforming qi. Clinically, it is marked by gastric stuffiness, fatigue, pale and lusterless complexion, emaciation, and so on. Another example concerns the mother-child relationship between the liver and the heart. Insufficiency of heart blood will give rise to deficiency of liver blood, resulting in heart-liver blood deficiency.

[**Previous Translation**] Illness of a child-organ may involve its mother organ; illness of the child stealing the mother-qi
[**Current Translation**] Illness of the child organ may involve the mother organ; child-organ disease affecting the mother-organ; Child-organ steals qi from its mother-organ; disorder of child-organ affecting mother-organ
[**Standard Translation**] Child organ affects mother organ.

Citations

- Insomnia occurs due to heart-qi deficiency caused by child organ affecting mother organ which gives rise to restlessness of the spirit and mind. (*Shishan's Case Records*)
- Pale complexion is the result of invasion by pathogenic qi when healthy qi is weakened due to child organ affecting mother organ. (*Principles Followed in Inspection Diagnosis*)
- Symptoms such as hoarse voice, sore throat, and cough with pink pus or blood occur due to kidney-yin deficiency which causes deficiency fire scorching lung metal, a pattern of child organ affecting mother organ. (*Wenzhai's Case Records*)

63. MŬBÌNG JÍ ZǏ 母病及子

Mother Organ Affects Child Organ

The term refers to the pathogenesis of mother organ affecting child organ in accordance with the generation among the five elements (i.e., zang-organs). For instance, the kidney pertains to water and the liver pertains to wood, and water generates wood; therefore, the kidney is the mother organ and the liver is the child organ. If a kidney disease affects the liver, it is described as mother organ affecting child organ. Clinically, it is marked by liver-yang hyperactivity—a result of kidney yin being too deficient to nourish liver wood, causing liver-yin deficiency, and thus making yin fail to restrict yang.

[Previous Translation] A MATERNAL DISEASE AFFECTING ITS OFFSPRING; Illness of a mother-organ may involve its child organ; diseased mother affecting the child; Illness of the mother organ affects the child one

[Current Translation] Disorders of the mother organ affecting the child organ; disorder of the mother-organ involving the child-organ; disorder of the mother-organ affecting its child-organ; illness of mother viscera affecting the child one; disorder of mother-organ affecting child-organ

[Standard Translation] Mother organ affects child organ.

Citations

- According to the five-element theory, the lung pertains to metal whose mother is earth. If the damp-heat in the stomach earth remains uncleared, it is bound to steam the lung in the upper energizer. This exemplifies the pattern of mother organ affecting child organ. (*Case Records of Four Doctors Selected by Liu Baozhi*)
- There is a pattern of mother organ affecting child organ. For example, lung disease can cause kidney disorders. (*True Transmission of Medical Principles*)
- Floating pulse indicates deficiency pattern, while wiry pulse suggests mother organ affecting child organ, which is the result of a kidney illness affecting the liver. (*Interpretation of Plain Conversation*)

64. JĪNSHÍ BÙ MÍNG 金实不鸣

A Solid Bell Cannot Ring

The term refers to the pathological change manifested as hoarse voice or even aphonia due to excess lung qi. The larynx is the gateway to the lung, the thoroughfare for the exiting and entering path of clear and turbid qi, and the main vocal organ. Lung qi causes the vocal cords in the larynx to vibrate and produce sound, and thus the lung governs sound. Physiologically, free and smooth flow of lung qi and sufficient lung yin jointly contribute to unobstructed breathing as well as loud and clear voice. Pathologically, if the lung is attacked by wind-cold or wind-heat, lung qi is unable to disperse normally, and symptoms such as hoarse voice, aphonia, itchy throat, and throat pain may occur. Since the lung pertains to metal in accordance with the five-element theory, the pathological change is described as the pattern that "a solid bell cannot ring."

[Previous Translation] DYSPHONIA DUE TO EXCESSIVE METAL; solid bell cannot be sounded; A broken bell does not ring

[Current Translation] A solid bell cannot ring; A solid bell cannot ring (hoarseness or dysphonia due to sthenia lung syndrome); hoarseness due to attack by external pathogenic factors; obstructed lung not functioning normally; muffled metal failing to sound

[Standard Translation] A solid bell cannot ring.

Citations

- In most cases, aphonia indicates lung diseases. It must be caused by acute illnesses as a result of binding constraint of pathogenic qi and ascending counterflow of qi, or by chronic illnesses as a result of exhaustion of fluids and blood.... This is described as the pattern that a solid bell cannot ring or a broken bell cannot ring. (*Comprehensive Medicine by Doctor Zhang Lu*)

- Coughing and hoarse voice are often the manifestations of the pattern that a solid bell cannot ring or a broken bell cannot ring. Patients with "a solid bell" should be treated with clearing and purging method, while those with "a broken bell" should be treated with supplementing therapy. The lung is the target for treatment in both cases. (*Key Link of Medicine*)

• Aphonia caused by coughing can be classified into four types: recently acquired, long-standing, deficiency, and excess. The recently acquired disorder often falls into the excess type, characterized by phlegm-fire obstruction and constraint described as the pattern that a solid bell cannot ring. The long-standing one often falls into the deficiency type, characterized by lung impairment and qi collapse described as the pattern that a broken bell cannot ring. (*Supplements for the Understanding of "Essential Prescriptions of the Golden Cabinet"*)

65. JĪNPÒ BÙ MÍNG 金破不鸣

A Broken Bell Cannot Ring

The term refers to the pathological change manifested as hoarse voice or even aphonia due to fluid consumption and the lack of moistening as a result of impairment and deficiency of lung qi and lung yin. According to the five-element theory, the lung pertains to metal. If lung qi is impaired and lung yin is insufficient, deficiency fire will scorch internally, causing symptoms such as faint voice, hoarseness or even aphonia, or dry and slightly painful throat, which is described as the pattern that "a broken bell cannot ring."

[**Previous Translation**] Dysphonia due to broken metal; Broken bell-metal cannot ring; A stuffed bell does not ring
[**Current Translation**] A broken gong does not sound; A broken bell does not sound (aphonia due to sthenia of pulmonary qi; sudden aphonia); hoarseness due to lung dysfunction; damaged lung not functioning normally; broken metal failing to sound
[**Standard Translation**] A broken bell cannot ring.

Citations

• Hoarse voice due to coughing is possibly caused by the constraint of phlegm-fire in the lung, which is described as the pattern that a solid bell cannot ring, or by the impairment of lung qi, which is described as the pattern that a broken bell cannot ring. (*A Complete Collection of Sore and Wound Treatment*)

- Impairment from consumptive disease and cough caused by endogenous pathogens, if not treated in time, will result in aphonia. This falls into the pattern that a broken bell cannot ring. (*Three-Character Medical Verses*)

66. SÌQÌ TIÁOSHÉN 四气调神

Regulating Life Activities According to Seasonal Changes

The term refers to the regulation of life activities in accordance with the climatic and phenological changes in the four seasons. Through the four seasons, the change of yin and yang is the root of life, characterized by sprouting in spring, growing in summer, harvesting in autumn, and storing in winter, a rule that human beings should comply with. Therefore, health preservation practice should be in concert with the climatic and phenological changes in the four seasons in order to maintain harmony between human life activities and natural seasonal changes. Specifically, in terms of everyday life, one should go to bed late and get up early in spring and summer months. To promote the growing, thriving, and dispersing of yang qi, one should also take strolls, stretch body, and moderately take part in outdoor activities. In autumn and winter time, to comply with the characteristics of elimination, concealment, and storage in nature, one should go to bed early, reduce activities proportionally, and avoid attack by external cold for the sake of astringing and storing yang qi. In terms of regulating spirit, it is preferable to relax and stay joyful in spring and summer in order to keep the smooth flow of qi, while it is better to keep peaceful and calm and maintain a restrained spirit in autumn and winter in order to store qi and spirit.

[**Previous Translation**] Regulating life activities according to natural changes in four seasons

[**Current Translation**] Regulating life activities according to seasonal changes

[**Standard Translation**] Regulating life activities according to seasonal changes

Citations

- Life activities should be regulated according to seasonal changes. Climate change can be deduced according to the theory of five circuits. The generation cycle resembles the relationship between mother and child; the restriction cycle, husband and wife. (*Classic of Holy Benevolence by Emperor Huizong of the Song Dynasty*)
- In Zhang's customary prescription, the addition and subtraction of medicinals are in accordance with the ascending or descending of yin and yang in the four seasons, which corresponds with the rule of "regulating life activities according to seasonal changes" in *Yellow Emperor's Internal Canon of Medicine.* (*Compendium of Chinese Medicine*)
- Regulating life activities according to seasonal changes is the key to preventing diseases and disorders by ancient Chinese sages. (*Effective Use of Established Formulas*)

67. TIÁNDÀN XŪWÚ 恬惔虚无

Placidity and Nothingness

The term means that one is calm and serene in mind, free from all desires and wants. Traditional Chinese medicine (TCM) emphasizes the relationship between emotional activities and physical well-being, and considers the internal organs and the refined essence transformed by them are the basis for the generation of emotions which, in turn, can have an effect on the human body. Therefore, it is important to cultivate spiritual health and maintain healthy qi in terms of health preservation and disease prevention in TCM. For spirit regulation, the top priority is to cultivate inner peace, abstaining from excessive desires. In other words, one should refrain from wants and desires, taking a humble and compatible attitude, being indifferent to fame or wealth, and being detached and refined to avoid experiencing negative emotions. In so doing, one can maintain a tranquil mind and have the spirit stored so that zang-fu organs as well as qi and blood can be regulated, free flow of qi can be attained, yin and yang can remain stable and compact, and body-spirit harmony can be achieved. Thus, one enjoys health and longevity.

[Previous Translation] /
[Current Translation] Calm and empty of cares and desires; tranquilized mind; indifferent to fame or gain; keep the mind pure and free from any avarice
[Standard Translation] Placidity and nothingness

Citations

- Keep placidity and nothingness (free from all desires and wants), and healthy qi in the body will be in harmony, spirit will remain inside. If so, how can diseases occur? (*Plain Conversation*)
- Thus, the sages never do anything against nature. They lead a placid life, free from all desires and wants, and feel at ease and happy. That is why they enjoy a happy and natural life span. (*Plain Conversation*)
- Placidity and nothingness refer to peace and quiet. Following the principle of peace and quiet in "Taoism," one can keep essential qi in the interior orderly and ward off pathogenic qi. (*Plain Conversation in Yellow Emperor's Internal Canon of Medicine Annotated by Wang Bing*)

68. ZHĪZHĬ BÙDÀI 知止不殆

Nothing Can Harm Who Stops in Time

The term means the person who knows when to stop will not invite danger. Traditional Chinese medicine emphasizes the relationship between emotions and health, believing that the excess of seven emotions can bring direct harm to the zang-fu organs, causing qi-movement disorder and subsequent diseases. To prevent negative emotions, it is very important for people to reduce desires and understand what is enough and when to stop to reduce conflict between needs and reality. If a person has excessive wants and needs, he/she is likely to experience depression, disappointment, sadness, anguish, and anger when his/her desires are not met, resulting in a disturbance of spirit, disorder of qi movement, and subsequent diseases. Only with least desires, peace of mind, and well-stored spirit can one achieve qi-blood harmony in the zang-fu organs, free flow of qi, strong immunity, and longevity.

[Previous Translation] /
[Current Translation] /
[Standard Translation] Nothing can harm who stops in time. In FLTRP version, it is stated in the explanatory notes that the translated version is borrowed from Arthur Waley.

Citations

- Fame or life, which is dearer? Life or wealth, which is more valuable? Between fame, wealth, and losing life, which is worse? Excessive love of fame costs greatly, and excessive hoard of goods invites catastrophic loss. Therefore, a person who is content with what he has will not be disgraced, and nothing can harm who stops in time. He is forever safe and secure. (*Lao Tseu*)
- One with higher status chooses to forget his privilege, while one with lower status is content with what he is. Neither is envious, and nothing can harm who stops in time. (*Original Decrees of Medicine*)

69. FǍ YÚ YĪNYÁNG 法于阴阳

Abiding by the Principle of Yin and Yang

Health preservation should be carried out in accordance with the principle of yin and yang in nature. According to *Yellow Emperor's Internal Canon of Medicine*, human life activities can be affected and restrained by climatic and phenological changes in the four seasons. Therefore, health should be preserved in accordance with the changes of yin and yang in nature to regulate physical functions, improve adaptability to environmental changes, and ward off pathogenic qi in the four seasons. The idea has since become an important guideline for health preservation and healthcare in later generations, and classics have never failed to include it throughout history.

[Previous Translation] According to Yin-Yang law
[Current Translation] Abiding by law of yin and yang; following the rule of yin and yang
[Standard Translation] Abiding by the principle of yin and yang

Citations

- The wise man in remote antiquity who knew ways of health preservation abode by the principle of yin and yang, regulated and nourished essential qi with *Shushu* (methods and techniques of health preservation). (*Plain Conversation*)
- Unpretentious and innocent nature is expounded first before the discussion on regulating and cultivating spirit. It is important to abide by the principle of yin and yang, and then regulate life activities in accordance with climatic and phenological changes in the four seasons. (*Attached Supplements to "Danxi's Mastery of Medicine"*)

70. HÉ YÚ SHÙSHÙ 和于术数

Regulating and Nourishing Essential Qi with Shushu

The term means using various appropriate methods to regulate and nourish essential qi. *Shushu* (术数, literally techniques and numbers) refers to the methods or techniques with which people predict human affairs, bring good fortune and outcast evil as well as speculate the fate and destiny of people and states based on scientific knowledge including astronomy, calendar, and musical temperament. It is conducted in accordance with the theories of "oneness of heaven and human" and "interaction between heaven and human" within the framework of yin-yang theory and the five-element theory. Based on a set of rules about numbers that are arbitrarily defined, various methods are used for the observation of noticeable phenomena in nature. *Shushu* herein refers to ways of health preservation such as *daoyin* and massage.

[Previous Translation] /
[Current Translation] Adjusting ways to cultivating health
[Standard Translation] Regulating and nourishing essential qi with *shushu*

Citations

- The wise man in remote antiquity who knew ways of health preservation abode by the principle of yin and yang, regulated and nourished essential qi with *shushu* (methods and techniques of health preservation). (*Plain Conversation*)

- *He* (和) means regulation, while *shushu* means ways of regulating and nourishing essential qi. (*Collective Annotations of Plain Conversation in Yellow Emperor's Internal Canon of Medicine*)
- *Shushu* is an umbrella term, including breathing and physical exercises such as inhalation and exhalation, massage, methods for preserving birth, growth, harvest, and storage discussed in the "Major Discussion on Regulation of Spirit According to the Changes of the Four Seasons." It also includes the concept that "yin is stable and yang is compact" in the "Discussion on Interrelationship between Life and Nature," "seven impairments and eight benefits" in the "Major Discussion on the Theory of Yin and Yang and the Corresponding Relationships Among All the Things in Nature," "long life with unfailing eyes and ears" in the "Basic State of Spirit" of *Spiritual Pivot*, and diets as well as lifestyles covered in the following part of this text. (*Annotations and Commentary of Plain Conversation in Yellow Emperor's Internal Canon of Medicine*)

71. QĪSǓN BĀYÌ 七损八益

Seven Impairments and Eight Benefits

The term refers to the seven harmful and eight beneficial ways of sex life in ancient times. According to the inscriptions on the bamboo slips, *Tian Xia Zhi Dao Tan* (*Discourse on the Utmost Method Under Heaven*), excavated in the Han Tombs at Mawangdui in Changsha, "The eight benefits are as follows: the first is regulating breathing; the second is promoting saliva; the third is understanding the proper time; the fourth is storing original qi; the fifth is harmonizing yin fluids; the sixth is accumulating essential qi; the seventh is maintaining abundance of essential qi, and the eighth is maintaining calm and balance. The seven impairments include internal blockage (suffering pain in sexual organs during the act), external leakage (perspiring during the act), exhaustion (consuming qi due to excessive engagement in the act), incompetence (impotence), vexation (feeling troubled and panting during the act), impasse (forcing oneself to engage in the act when the partner has no desire), and waste (performing the act in haste)."[1]

[Previous Translation] INSUFFICIENCY OF SEVEN AND TONIFICATION OF EIGHT; seven harmful methods and eight favorable techniques in sexual life
[Current Translation] Sevenfold impairment and eightfold benefit; seven ills and eight benefits; seven impairments and eight benefits
[Standard Translation] Seven impairments and eight benefits

Citations

- Yin and yang can be harmonized if the precepts of seven impairments and eight benefits are followed. Otherwise, people will age prematurely. (*Plain Conversation*)
- Understanding seven impairments and eight benefits will help prevent yin from predominance and yang from deficiency, and hence the harmony between yin and yang can be achieved. (*Explanation of Unresolved Issues in the "Plain Conversation"*)
- One can prudently maintain his congenital qi if he does not marry before age twenty and sticks to the precepts of seven impairments and eight benefits advanced by the sages. (*Consistent Medical Principles*)

72. YĪNSHÌ LÌDǍO 因势利导

Treatment in Accordance with the Tendency of Pathological Changes

The term refers to making things develop in a direction favorable to the accomplishment of goals in accordance with their trends in development. In traditional Chinese medicine, it is important to consider all factors in the treatment of diseases including the course, site, and characteristics of diseases and to comply with the theory of waxing and waning of yin and

---

[1] English translation is based on: Douglas Wile (1992). Art of the Bedchamber: The Chinese Sexual Yoga Classics Including Women's Solo Meditation Texts. New York: State University of New York Press. p. 81.

yang as well as the principle of qi and blood circulation in the zang-fu organs. It is also important to grasp the best time, to fully mobilize and exploit the physiological mechanism and human body's capacity of "spontaneous harmonization of yin and yang" in fighting, dispelling, and curing diseases, to adopt the most appropriate therapy for treatment, and to promote automatic self-regulation so that the balance of yin and yang, qi, and blood can be restored. For example, according to different conditions of the diseases located in the upper, lower, exterior, or interior part of the human body, different therapies such as emesis, purgation, and relieving superficies can be used respectively to eliminate a disease in a simplest and fastest way. In doing so, no or less healthy qi is impaired and best outcomes can be achieved at the lowest cost.

[**Previous Translation**] Treatment in accordance with the tendency of pathological changes
[**Current Translation**] Treatment in accordance with tendency of pathological changes
[**Standard Translation**] Treatment in accordance with the tendency of pathological changes

Citations

- In terms of treating diarrhea ... Pathogenic qi will be enhanced if qi-supplementing method is used, and fire clearing may worsen symptoms of diarrhea. Only with the treatment in accordance with the tendency of pathological changes can such an intractable condition be relieved. (*Secret Records in Stone Room*)
- Patients with deep pulse have pathogenic qi inside their bodies. It would be relatively easier to treat them with purgative method to dispel pathogens, which fits with the treatment in accordance with the tendency of pathological changes. (*Understanding of "Essential Prescriptions of the Golden Cabinet"*)
- The outbreak of malaria in the morning is due to the upper location of pathogens, which is in the yang phase. It should be treated in accordance with the tendency of pathological changes, administering *Xiao Chaihu* Decoction (Minor Bupleurum Decoction) with the addition of *zhiqiao* (*Fructus Aurantii*, orange fruit) and *jiegeng* (*Radix Platycodonis*, platycodon root). (*Comprehensive Medicine by Doctor Zhang Lu*)

73. YĬ PÍNG WÉI QĪ 以平为期

Achieving Yin-yang Balance

The term means the goal of the treatment is to restore the relative balance between yin and yang in humans. In traditional Chinese medicine, physiological activities should work well to retain a healthy state if dynamic balance could be maintained among the zang-fu organs and tissues as well as between the person and the environment. Otherwise, diseases would occur. Therefore, holistically speaking, treating a disease is to rectify deviations and to coordinate the relationship between internal and external environment in order to keep a balance. Apart from adjusting the preponderance or deficiency of yin or yang to bring them back to normal, disharmony between qi and blood, zang-fu organs as well as disturbance in ascending and descending should be regulated to restore balance.

[Previous Translation]
[Current Translation] /
[Standard Translation] Achieving yin-yang balance

Citations

- To achieve yin-yang balance, careful observation on their location should be made of yin and yang before regulation. (*Plain Conversation*).
- The medicine warm in property should be used in treating those diseases cold in nature and taken when it is hot. The purpose is to achieve yin-yang balance and not to overuse the medicine, which is the key to the treatment. (*Book for Saving Lives*).
- The focus of the treatment is purging excess and supplementing deficiency, with the purpose of achieving yin-yang balance in humans. (*Confucian's Duties to Their Parents*).

74. SĪWÀI CHUĂINÈI 司外揣内

Judging Internal Condition by Observing External Manifestations

The term, also known as "knowing the inside through the outside," refers to the cognitive method via which people judge internal condition by observing external manifestations. According to the "Gaozi Part II" of *Mencius*, "the inside must be mirrored in the outside," denoting that people in ancient times had realized the interrelationship between essence and phenomenon and the internal changes could be manifested in external aspects. Therefore, by observing external manifestations, internal mechanism of changes can be understood up to a certain point. Through the observation on and identification of life phenomena, traditional Chinese medicine witnesses the development of perceptual cognition. It discovers and summarizes the fixed relationship between the nature of a living thing and its external condition. The concept is then established and the study of "manifestation" is completed, which is part of the work involved in "judging internal condition by observing external manifestations." The concept is further developed by identification and reasoning, reaching the level of "judging internal condition." "Judging" is essentially the logical thinking process from manifestation observation to concept development, involving making judgment and reasoning. Therefore, "judging internal condition by observing external manifestations" denotes the means and way of thinking adopted to understand the law of life at the "manifestation-condition" level in humans.

[**Previous Translation**] /
[**Current Translation**] Judging the inside by observation of the outside; predict the interior by inspecting the exterior; judging the inside from observation of the outside; inspecting exterior to predict interior
[**Standard Translation**] Judging internal condition by observing external manifestations

Citations

- From the external perspective, internal pathological changes can be judged by examining external manifestations of the patient. In turn, the external manifestations can be deduced by understanding the internal disorders of the zang-fu organs. (*Spiritual Pivot*)

- Observing external manifestations can provide health information of one's zang-fu organs and help predict the diseases that may occur. (*Spiritual Pivot*)
- By comparing normal conditions of themselves with abnormal conditions of patients and by examining external manifestations, doctors gain an understanding of internal pathological changes. These are the methods they use to identify predominance and/or insufficiency of certain aspects. (*Plain Conversation*)

75. JIÀNWĒI ZHĪZHÙ 见微知著

Deducing Significant Changes from Subtle Signs

Subtle signs could indicate significant changes and outcomes that may occur. It figuratively means predicting the big from the small. According to traditional Chinese medicine, *wei* (微, subtle or tiny) refers to small, local changes in body parts and *zhu* (著, significant) refers to obvious, overall state of the body. The term means that local and minor changes can indicate the physiological and pathological information of the whole body, that is, the overall condition is mirrored in local subtle changes as the diseases in whole body can be manifested in many aspects. By examining these subtle changes, the overall condition can be determined. Examinations of pulse, face, tongue, and ears are the applications of this principle in practice.

[Previous Translation] /
[Current Translation] /
[Standard Translation] Deducing significant changes from subtle signs

Citations

- Treating a disease when it occurs is what the inferior doctor does. The superior doctor could deduce significant changes from subtle signs and would nip potential risks in the bud. (*Medical Understanding*)
- If you can deduce significant changes when noticing subtle signs of a disease, will you repeat the mistakes of your predecessors? (*Yu Chang's Case Records and Treatments*)

- The ancients put prevention first instead of treating patients when they fall ill. Those who understand this principle could predict significant changes of the diseases when noticing subtle signs; therefore, regulating and cultivating health is the best strategy. (*Case Records of Jingxiang Mansion*)

76. YǏ CHÁNG HÉNG BIÀN 以常衡变

Discerning Changes by Measuring Against the Normal

Based on an understanding of the normal state, one can differentiate and discover abnormal changes such as excess or inadequacy. *Chang* (常, normal) refers to the healthy physiological state; *bian* (变, change) refers to the abnormal pathological state. According to traditional Chinese medicine (TCM) diagnosis, emphasis should be first laid upon knowing the healthy state of average people and taking the "normal" as the standard to identify differences and the disease. According to the "Discussion on Qi Manifestation in a Healthy Person" of *Plain Conversation*, for example, excess and/or deficiency of a disease could be determined based on the relationship between the respiration and pulsing of a healthy person. For a healthy individual, the pulse beats four times in a cycle of exhalation and inhalation. If the ratio exceeds it, it is rapid pulse; if it is fewer than four times, it is slow pulse. Guided by the principle of discerning changes by measuring against the normal, TCM practitioners examine the complexion and the tongue of patients.

[**Previous Translation**] /
[**Current Translation**] /
[**Standard Translation**] Discerning changes by measuring against the normal

Citations

- Healthy individuals are those who are not ill. The respiratory rate of a healthy individual is usually used as the criterion to measure the pulse conditions of sick people. Doctors are healthy individuals, so they can regulate their rate of breathing to examine the pulse beats of their patients. (*Plain Conversations*)

- The principle of pulse-taking is to discern changes by measuring against the normal pulse. Normal pulse conditions should be well understood so that abnormalities can be identified. (*Jingyue's Complete Works*)
- When complexion, pulse condition, and other manifestations are in consistency, it is considered normal; if not, it is considered abnormal. By understanding the normal and abnormal states of the body, the doctor could diagnose the diseases. (*Principles Followed in Inspection Diagnosis*)

77. YĪN FĀ ZHĪ SHÒU 因发知受

Disease Manifestations Help Determine the Cause

Doctors should determine the pathogenic factors, that is, wind, cold, summer-heat, dampness, dryness, and fire, based on the manifested disease pattern rather than climate change, temperature, or humidity. *Fa* (发, manifestation) refers to the signs and symptoms of the pattern that occur. *Shou* (受, receiving) refers to the pathogenic qi that one is affected and the responses that one's body makes. Whether the disease occurs or not after various pathogenic qi affects the body depends on the result of the fight between healthy qi and pathogenic qi. The nature of pathogenic qi is mainly determined through the differentiation of a pattern. For example, when the weather suddenly changes, not everyone will be affected by external pathogens. Whether and by what kind of pathogenic qi one is affected are mainly determined by one's body's ability and condition to cope with pathogens, and these must be diagnosed according to the signs and symptoms manifested in the body. This method of identifying the cause is also described as "examining symptoms to identify the cause," that is, to understand the internal mechanism and the nature of disease development by examining the signs and symptoms.

[**Previous Translation**] Assess the patterns and seek the cause; seek the cause from patterns identified [Note: It refers to examining symptoms to identify the cause (shěn zhèng qiú yīn 审症求因)].

[**Current Translation**] Seeking the cause from symptoms; determining the cause of the disease according to the clinical manifestations; differentiating syndrome to identify cause; identification of cause according to syndrome differentiation [Note: They refer to examining symptoms to identify the cause (shěn zhèng qiú yīn 审症求因)].

[**Standard Translation**] Disease manifestations help determine the cause.

Citations

- It is hard to surmise what kind of external pathogen affects the human body before the onset of a disease is shown. It can be identified after the disease occurs. Manifestations could help determine the cause of the disease. (*Tracing Cold Damage to Its Source*)
- An examination of the pulse and other symptoms can help identify the cause of the disease and the treatment should be given in accordance with the pattern. (*Treatise on Cold Damage*)

78. SÌZHĚN HÉCĀN 四诊合参

Synthesis of the Four Diagnostic Methods

The four equally important diagnostic methods are used for cross-reference, including inspection, listening and smelling, inquiry, and pulse-taking and palpation. The collected information of the diseases should be considered thoroughly in order to make an accurate diagnosis. Disease is a complex process and its clinical manifestations can be reflected in various aspects and may change from time to time. The four diagnostic methods are adopted to understand the diseases and help collect the relevant information from different perspectives, each with its unique technique and value. They cannot replace each other. If only one single method is used, it will inevitably lead to the one-sidedness of data collection, which will affect the accuracy of diagnosis. Therefore, in order to obtain comprehensive, accurate, and detailed clinical data, it is more than necessary to emphasize the combined use of the four diagnostic methods and they should supplement one another.

[Previous Translation] Comprehensive analysis by the four examination methods; DEDUCTION BY THE FOUR DIAGNOSTIC TECHNIQUES; comprehensive analysis by four methods of examination; comprehensive diagnosis by four methods; correlate all four examination; correlation of all four examinations

[Current Translation] Comprehensive analysis of the data obtained by the four diagnostic techniques; comprehensive consideration of the four examinations; synthesis of four diagnostic method; comprehensive diagnosis by four methods; comprehensive analysis of the data obtained from the four examinations; synthesis of the four diagnostics; correlation of all four examinations; comprehensive analysis of four examinations [**Standard Translation**] Synthesis of the four diagnostic methods

Citations

- Examination of facial complexion in terms of freshness or turbidity could help identify yin or yang property of the disease; examination in terms of dark or light color could help determine deficiency or excess nature of the disease. The synthesis of the four diagnostic methods cannot go wrong, can it? (*Principles Followed in Inspection Diagnosis*)
- Superior doctors should value all four diagnostic methods when they aspire to understand the disease comprehensively. (*Binhu Study on Pulses*)

79. SĀNBÙ JIǓHÒU 三部九候

Three Sections and Nine Manifestations

The term refers to the pulse-taking method of feeling the arterial pulse of the head, hands, and feet to diagnose diseases. It was first described in the "Discussion on Three Sections and Nine Manifestations" of *Plain Conversation*. The arteries of the three sections, that is, head (upper), hand (middle), and foot (lower), are palpated and each section is further divided into three subsections, namely, heaven, human, and earth, making nine sections altogether. The upper-section heaven refers to the temporal arteries on both sides, which can indicate the pain in the forehead and temples; the upper-section human, the anterior auricular artery, can reveal the condition of the eyes and the ears; the upper-section earth, the cheek arteries, can manifest the condition of the mouth and teeth. The middle-section heaven refers to the artery of the Lung Meridian of Hand-*taiyin*, where the condition of lung qi can be manifested; the middle-section human refers to the artery of the Heart Meridian of Hand-*shaoyin*, where the condition of heart qi can be detected; the middle-section earth refers to the artery of the Large Intestine Meridian of Hand-*yangming*, where the condition of chest qi can be revealed. The lower-section heaven is the artery of the Liver Meridian of Foot-*jueyin*, which can reflect the condition of liver qi; the lower-section human refers to the artery of the Spleen

Meridian of Foot-*taiyin* or the Stomach Meridian of Foot-*yangming*, which can indicate the condition of spleen qi and stomach qi; the lower-section earth is the artery of the Kidney Meridian of Foot-*shaoyin*, which can reveal the condition of kidney qi. Later generations adopt *cunkou* diagnostic method (see the following entry), taking *cun* (寸), *guan* (关), and *chi* (尺) as the three sections for pulse-taking. Then pulse-taking at each section is divided into three different aspects according to the force, that is, light, medium, and heavy, thus making a total of nine manifestations. This is also described as three sections and nine manifestations.

[**Previous Translation**] Three regions and their nine subdivisions for pulse-feeling; three regions and nine modes; three regions and nine locations for pulse feeling; three portions and nine pulse-takings; three positions and nine indicators

[**Current Translation**] Three portions and nine pulse-taking; nine readings of three sections; three regions, three portions (for pulse taking); three portions and nine positions for pulse-taking; nine readings on three sections; three positions and nine indicators; three positions and nine pulse-takings

[**Standard Translation**] Three sections and nine manifestations

Citations

- Therefore, there are three sections for pulse-taking in the human body and each section is divided into three subsections, which are examined to determine prognosis, diagnose diseases, and relieve deficiency and/or excess to remove diseases. (*Plain Conversation*)
- Irregular and disharmonic pulse signifies impending diseases. If all the nine manifestations on three sections are in disharmony, it indicates impending death. (*Plain Conversation*)
- The *cunkou* diagnostic method means the examination of three sections and nine manifestations. What does each mean? Here is the answer: the three sections refer to *cun, guan,* and *chi*; the nine manifestations refer to the results obtained by taking pulse using three different levels of force, i.e., light, medium, and heavy, respectively. (*Canon of Difficult Issues*)

80. CÙNKǑU ZHĚNFǍ 寸口诊法

Cunkou *Diagnostic Method*

The term refers to the diagnostic method of feeling the pulse at the radial artery in the medial side of the styloid, through which the doctor could determine the physiological and pathological states of a human body. A prominent bone, that is, styloid process of the radius, marks the section. The medial part of it is *guan* (关); in the front of *guan* (to the wrist) is *cun* (寸), and at the back of *guan* (to the elbow) is *chi* (尺). There are three sections on each hand and therefore six in total. At the sections of *cun, guan,* and *chi,* pulse can be taken respectively with three different levels of force, that is, light, medium, and heavy. Each section is believed to correspond to one of the zang-fu organs. *Cun* on the left hand corresponds to the heart and *cun* on the right hand, the lung, including the parts above the chest and the head as well. *Guan* on the left hand corresponds to the liver and the gallbladder; *Guan* on the right hand, the spleen and stomach, including the parts between the diaphragm and the umbilicus. *Chi* on both hands corresponds to the kidney, including the parts in between the umbilicus and the feet. Instead of using *cun, guan,* and *chi,* one can examine the conditions of the zang-fu organs according to the applied force in three levels, that is, light, medium, and heavy. For example, on the left hand, light force, medium force, and heavy force are used to identify the condition of the heart, the liver, and the kidney, respectively. On the right hand, they are used to identify the condition of the lung, the spleen, and the kidney (life gate), respectively.

[**Previous Translation**] /
[**Current Translation**] Wrist pulse-taking method; wrist pulse-taking method; wrist pulse-taking method; wrist pulse-taking method; *cun* pulse-taking method
[**Standard Translation**] *Cunkou* diagnostic method

Citations

- In the discourse on pulse-taking, examination of facial complexion, and inspecting the skin from the elbow to the wrist, the statement refers to *cunkou* diagnostic method. (*Bianque's Canon of Difficult Issues on Pulse-taking*)
- It is ingenious to only adopt *cunkou* diagnostic method at present. (*Classified Classic*)

81. BIÀNZHÈNG LÙNZHÌ 辨证论治

Pattern Differentiation and Treatment

The term refers to the thinking process and the practice of differentiating the patterns based on the collected data and formulating the corresponding treatment plan in accordance with the theory of traditional Chinese medicine (TCM). It involves two stages: pattern differentiation and treatment. The former means collecting data as well as signs and symptoms through the four diagnostic methods (inspection, listening and smelling, inquiry, and pulse-taking and palpation) and making a comprehensive analysis of information to differentiate the cause, nature, and location of the disease and then to identify the relationship between pathogenic qi and healthy qi under the guidance of TCM theory. One is expected to eventually generalize the data to a pattern of certain nature. Such is the logical thinking process of understanding the disease from the perspective of body's responses. Analyzing clinical manifestations helps one identify their internal relationships, based on which the nature of the disease can be determined at a certain stage. The latter involves determining the corresponding treatment principle and methods based on pattern differentiation and opting for appropriate therapies to remove diseases.

[**Previous Translation**] BIANZHEN LUNZHI (PLANNING TREATMENT ACCORDING TO DIAGNOSIS); selection of treatment based on the differential diagnosis; treatment based on syndrome differentiation; identify patterns and determine treatment; determine treatment by patterns identified; diagnosis and treatment based on the overall analysis of signs and symptoms; treatment with syndrome differentiation

[**Current Translation**] Selection of treatment according to differential diagnosis; treatment based on syndrome differentiation; syndrome differentiation and treatment; pattern identification; syndrome differentiation and treatment; pattern identification and treatment

[**Standard Translation**] Pattern differentiation and treatment

Citations

- How could the disease be cured if the doctor did not know the theory of six qi (wind, cold, summer-heat, dampness, dryness, and fire) or the principle of treating diseases based on pattern differentiation? (*Medical Warnings*)
- Pattern differentiation and treatment, as the tradition of study style inherited from the master to the apprentice in the Han and Tang dynasties, is indeed profound and can be the eternal principle to follow. (*Fair Interpretation of Wind Stroke*)
- Zhang Zhongjing wrote books to expound his theories.... (He) was the first physician to advance the idea of pattern differentiation and treatment for later scholars to abide by. (*Tracing Cold Damage to Its Source*)

82. TÓNGBÌNG YÌZHÌ 同病异治

Different Treatments for the Same Disease

The term means that the same disease should be treated with different approaches according to different patterns manifested at different stages or resulting from variations in such factors as geography, climate, and body constitution. Take measles for example. The treatment should vary according to the pathological development at different stages. In the early stage, rashes are not fully developed and the treatment should be resolving superficies to promote eruption. In the mid-stage, lung heat is always prominent, so it is important to clear the lung. In the late stage, remaining heat is always present and impairs lung yin and stomach yin, which requires nourishing yin and clearing heat.

[**Previous Translation**] Treating the same disease with different methods; different treatments for the same disease

[**Current Translation**] Treating the same disease with different methods; different treatments for the same disease

[**Standard Translation**] Different treatments for the same disease

Citations

- Neck carbuncle due to the stagnation of qi can be treated with acupuncture to disperse qi. Cases with formed pus due to predominance of qi and coagulation of blood can be treated with stone needle to remove static blood. Such treatments are known as different treatments for the same disease. (*Plain Conversation*)
- It is cold in the northwest, so the treatment should concentrate on dissipating cold and clearing interior heat; it is warm in the southeast, so the treatment should focus on astringing the leakage of yang qi and dissipating interior cold by warming. This is described as different treatments for the same disease. (*Plain Conversation*)

83. YÌBÌNG TÓNGZHÌ 异病同治

Same Treatment for Different Diseases

The term means that different diseases could be treated with the same method when they manifest the same or similar pathological change or disease pattern in their development. For example, such diseases as chronic enteritis, nephritis, and asthma could be treated with the same method of warming and tonifying kidney yang since all of them show the pathological change of kidney yang deficiency in their progression.

[**Previous Translation**] Treat the different diseases with the same method; treating different diseases with same therapy, treating different diseases with the same method; like treatment of unlike disease; the same treatment for different diseases

[**Current Translation**] Treating different diseases with the same therapeutic principle; same treatment for different diseases; treating different diseases with the same therapy; treating different diseases with the same method

[**Standard Translation**] Same treatment for different diseases

Citations

- This disease is like the following conditions: pathogenic qi of the febrile disease remains dormant in the *shaoyin* meridian, pathogenic heat consumes stomach yin, and pathogenic fire invades the pericardium. Therefore, all of them could be treated with the same method. (*Comprehensive Medicine by Doctor Zhang Lu*)

- For these diseases, either the rule of different treatments for the same disease or the principle of same treatment for different diseases should be followed. (*Rules and Principles of Moxibustion*)

84. HÁNYĪN HÁNYÒNG 寒因寒用

Treating Cold with Cold

The term refers to one of the paradoxical treatments, meaning using cold-natured medicinals to treat the diseases with cold signs and symptoms. This method is applicable to relieving the pattern of true heat with pseudo-cold manifestations due to exuberant interior heat preventing yang qi from reaching out to the skin. Take heat syncope for example. On the one hand, internal yang heat is predominant and pathogenic heat is hidden deep inside, showing symptoms of interior heat such as high fever, aversion to heat, vexation, thirst with a desire for cold drinks, dark urine, and rapid pulse. On the other hand, the extremely predominant interior heat prevents yang qi from flowing outward and causes pseudo-cold manifestations such as reversal cold of the limbs and deep pulse. In this case, medicinals cold and/or cool in nature should be used to clear the internal heat to remove the root cause of the disease, thus having the pseudo-cold symptoms relieved accordingly.

[**Previous Translation**] Treating the pseudo-cold diseases with drugs of cold nature; treating cold with cold; using medicines of cold nature to treat pseudo-cold syndrome

[**Current Translation**] Using drugs of cold nature to treat pseudo-cold syndrome; using cold for cold; treating false cold syndrome with cold herbs; using herbs of cold nature to treat pseudo-cold syndrome; using cold when the cause is cold; treat cold with cold; treating cold with cold

[**Standard Translation**] Treating cold with cold

Citations

- Treat heat with heat, and treat cold with cold.... To cure a disease, the cause must be made clear first. (*Plain Conversation*)
- Or treat cold with cold; treat heat with heat. Either is appropriate if treatment is given in accordance with specific conditions. (*Compendium of Pediatrics*)

85. RÈYĪN RÈYÒNG 热因热用

Treating Heat with Heat

The term refers to one of the paradoxical treatments, meaning using medicinal of hot nature to treat the diseases with heat manifestations. Take *shaoyin* disease with excessive internal yin-cold for example. Its clinical manifestations include diarrhea with undigested food, reversal cold of the extremities, as well as faint and impalpable pulse. However, pseudo-heat signs and symptoms such as "red complexion" and "no aversion to cold" can be present due to exuberant yin repelling yang. Therefore, *Tongmai Sini* Decoction (Decoction for Treating Cold Limbs by Promoting Vessels) of warm-hot nature is adopted in compliance with the exterior heat but in conflict with the root cause of yin cold. Another example is the qi-deficiency pattern with fever. Due to the deficiency of yang qi of the spleen and the stomach, the essence derived from food and drinks fails to ascend but descends instead to the lower energizer and transforms into yin fire which disturbs upwards and causes fever. *Buzhong Yiqi* Decoction (Decoction for Tonifying Middle Energizer and Boosting Qi) of sweet-warm property should be used to ascend spleen yang (qi) and raise the sinking essential qi, which is described as removing fever with medicinals sweet in flavor and warm in property. This is also an example of treating heat with heat.

[**Previous Translation**] Treat the pseudo-heat syndrome with drugs of hot nature; treating heat with heat; treating pseudo-heat diseases with drugs of hot nature; using herbs of hot nature to treat pseudo-heat syndrome

[**Current Translation**] Using warm-natured drugs to treat pseudo-heat syndrome; using heat for heat; treating pseudo-heat syndrome with hot therapy; using heat when the cause is heat; treat heat with heat

[**Standard Translation**] Treating heat with heat

Citations

- Treat heat with heat, and treat cold with cold.... To cure a disease, the cause must be made clear first. (*Plain Conversation*)

- Some people question why *Buzhong Yiqi* Decoction (Decoction for Tonifying Middle Energizer and Boosting Qi) could treat fever. It is surprising that they know nothing about the principle of treating heat with heat, i.e., medicine of warm nature could relieve fever. (*Guide to Saving Yang*)

86. TŌNGYĪN TŌNGYÒNG 通因通用

Treating the Flowing by Promoting Flow

The term refers to one of the paradoxical treatments, meaning treating the excess pattern with "flowing" disorders such as diarrhea using medicinals of unblocking function. This method is applicable to relieving diarrhea due to the internal retention of excessive pathogenic factors. For example, the pattern of "heat fecaloma with watery discharge" characterized by internal dryness-heat retention and diarrhea should be treated with *Chengqi* Decoction (Decoction for Purging Digestive Qi) to relieve dryness excess. According to *Treatise on Cold Damage*, "*Shaoyin* disease, characterized by spontaneous watery diarrhea of a greenish color, manifests pain below the heart. If the mouth is parched, purgative method can be used. *Da Cheng Qi* Decoction (Major Decoction for Purging Digestive Qi) is appropriate." Other examples are as follows. When there is food retention in the stomach and intestines causing stomachache, borborygmus, and diarrhea with a foul stench of rotten eggs, it requires promoting digestion and purging stagnation. When there is metrorrhagia or metrostaxis with blood clots due to blood stasis and abdominal pain which is aggravated by pressure, or postpartum blood stagnation and lochiorrhea, it needs promoting blood circulation to remove stagnation. In terms of dampness-heat accumulation in the urinary bladder causing frequent, urgent, and painful urination, the method of clearing heat, draining dampness, and relieving stranguria should be adopted. For the dysentery due to dampness-heat accumulation in the large intestine which results in serious diarrhea for more than ten times a day, the treatment should be clearing heat to remove intestinal obstruction and regulating qi to promote blood circulation instead of astringing.

[**Previous Translation**] Treat the diarrhetic diseases with cathartics; treating diarrhea by purgation; treating diarrhea with cathartics; using purgative method to treat unconfinedness; treating the stopped by stopping; treating diarrhea with purgatives

[**Current Translation**] Treating discharging disease with purgatives; opening for the opened; using dredging method when the cause is incontinence; treat diarrhea with purgative; treating the unstopped by unstopping; treating incontinent syndrome with dredging method; treat dredging with dredging

[**Standard Translation**] Treating the flowing by promoting flow

Citations

- The Yellow Emperor asked: "What does paradoxical treatment mean?" Qibo answered: "Paradoxical treatment means treating heat with heat, treating cold with cold, treating the blocked by blocking, and treating the flowing by promoting flow." (*Plain Conversation*)
- The method of "treating the flowing by promoting flow" should be used in the case of tenesmus with frequent visits to the toilet but have difficulty in defecation. (*Confucians' Duties to Their Parents*)
- In terms of dysentery... at its onset, original qi is not deficient so purgative method should be used, which is treating the flowing by promoting flow. (*Danxi's Mastery of Medicine*)

87. SĀIYĪN SĀIYÒNg 塞因塞用

Treating the Blocked by Blocking

The term refers to one of the paradoxical treatments, meaning treating the deficient pattern with obstructive signs and symptoms by using tonifying medicine. This method is applicable to relieving obstructive patterns due to the hypofunction of zang-fu organs caused by insufficiency of yin, yang, qi, and blood. For example, amenorrhea due to insufficiency of essential qi and deficiency of thoroughfare vessel and conception vessel should be treated by replenishing kidney qi and nourishing the liver, the kidney, and blood to regulate menstruation. In terms of deficient constipation, it requires nourishing blood and moistening dryness in the case of blood deficiency; reinforcing qi to invigorate spleen yang in the case of qi deficiency causing inability to transport essence; warming yang qi in the case of yang deficiency; or nourishing fluids and supplementing yin to promote body-fluid production and bowel movement in the case of fluid deficiency. As for dysuria, it requires supplementing lung qi to restore its regulation of waterway in the case of insufficiency of lung qi causing disorder of regulating water passage; supplementing middle-qi to ascend spleen qi and descend turbid yin in the case of spleen-qi sinking causing failure to ascend the clear and descend the turbid; or warming kidney yang and transforming qi to promote diuresis in the case of kidney-yang deficiency and life-gate-fire decline leading to qi-transformation disorder of the urinary bladder.

[**Previous Translation**] Treat the pseudo-obstructive disease with tonics; TREATING OBSTRUCTION BY TONIFICATION; treating the obstruction-syndrome with tonics; using tonify method to treat obstructive syndrome; treating the stopped by stopping; treating obstruction by tonification; treating obstructive syndrome with nourishing therapy

[**Current Translation**] Treating obstructive diseases by tonification; filling for the stuffed; using blockage when the cause is blockage; treat stuffiness with tonic; treating the stopped by stopping; treating obstructive syndrome with dredging method; treat block with block

[**Standard Translation**] Treating the blocked by blocking

Citations

- Treat the blocked by blocking, and treat the flowing by promoting flow. To cure a disease, the cause must be made clear first. (*Plain Conversation*)
- Treat the blocked by blocking. For example, when healthy qi in the lower energizer is deficient and that in the middle energizer stagnates, promoting the flow of qi to relieve abdominal distension may worsen the deficiency of healthy qi in the lower energizer.... Instead, greatly reinforcing healthy qi in the lower energizer can help with qi restoration, which relieves fullness in the middle energizer. (*Essentials of the Internal Canon of Medicine*)

88. BIĀOBĚN HUĂNJÍ 标本缓急

Branch, Root, the Non-acute, and the Acute

The term refers to the way of thinking that appropriate therapeutic methods should be determined based on the differentiation of primary factors and secondary factors, the branch and the root, the minor and the major, as well as the non-acute and the acute and on the analysis of their relationships among the various factors in complicated and variable patterns. *Biao* and *ben*, literally referring to the branch and the root of a plant, can be figuratively used to explain the relationship between the primary and the secondary factors. Therefore, as a pair of contrary concepts, they have multiple connotations in different contexts. For example, with respect to healthy qi (root), pathogenic qi is regarded as the branch in the disease development. In the relation between disease cause and symptoms, the latter is the branch. In terms of disease sequence, the old or primary disease is the root and the new or secondary disease is the branch. Finally, as for diseased sites, the internal zang-fu organs are viewed as the roots and the exterior manifestations are the branches. In terms of treating complex patterns, it is advisable to identify the primary conflict or the primary aspect of the conflict, distinguishing the primary from the secondary, the major from the minor, as well as the acute from the non-acute to cure diseases. Generally, in acute and severe cases, either the branch or the root should be treated first if it is acute; if both are acute, they should be treated at the same time. In non-acute cases, the root should be treated first or both the root and the branch are treated at the same time.

[**Previous Translation**] /
[**Current Translation**] /
[**Standard Translation**] Branch, root, the non-acute, and the acute

Citations

- If the doctors did not know the principle of the branch and the root as well as that of the non-acute and the acute, it is inevitable to misdiagnose the diseases and bring harm to patients. (*Treatise on Seasonal Diseases*)

- If the disease is complicated, one should differentiate between the root and the branch as well as the non-acute and the acute before giving corresponding treatment. (*Medical Understanding*)
- In the case of disease transformation, it is advisable to differentiate between the branch and the root as well as the non-acute and the acute. The treatment sequence and whether to treat one disease only or two or more simultaneously should be made clear. Medicinals for treating both the root cause and symptoms (the branch) should be used. If things are dealt with in order, various diseases can be relieved. (*Treatise on the Origin and Development of Medicine*)

89. FÚZHÈNG QŪXIÉ 扶正祛邪

Reinforcing Healthy Qi and Eliminating Pathogenic Qi

The term refers to one of the fundamental therapeutic principles in traditional Chinese medicine. Reinforcing healthy qi means improving the anti-pathogenic ability and promoting rehabilitation by supporting healthy qi and enhancing body constitution, including various methods such as boosting qi, nourishing blood, enriching yin, warming yang, supplementing essence, fortifying the zang-fu organs, and so on. It is applicable to the treatment of various deficiency patterns caused by deficient healthy qi. Eliminating pathogenic qi means inhibiting hyperactive pathological reactions and reducing pathological damage by eliminating pathogenic factors and resolving internally generated toxins, including methods such as promoting sweat, inducing vomiting, purgation, clearing heat, relieving food stagnation, dispelling wind, draining dampness, resolving phlegm, and invigorating blood to dissolve stasis, and so on. It is applicable to the treatment of various excess patterns caused by excessive pathogenic qi. Reinforcing healthy qi and eliminating pathogenic qi are opposite but complementary methods, forming an interdependent relationship. When healthy qi is enhanced, it will assist the body to expel pathogenic qi, which is described as "with strengthened healthy qi, pathogenic qi will recede automatically." On the other hand, when pathogenic qi is eliminated, healthy qi will be protected from further impairment, which is described as "with pathogenic qi being dispelled, healthy qi is safeguarded naturally."

[**Previous Translation**] Support the healthy energy and eliminate the evil factors; REINFORCING BODY RESISTANCE TO ELIMINATE PATHOGENS; supporting healthy energy to eliminate evils; strengthening the genuine qi to eliminate the evil qi

[**Current Translation**] Supporting the body resistance (扶正); supporting vital qi (扶正); supporting the healthy and eliminating the evil; strengthening healthy qi to eliminate pathogenic factors; reinforcing the healthy qi to eliminate pathogenic qi; reinforce the healthy and eliminate the pathogenic; strengthening vital qi to eliminate pathogenic factor

[**Standard Translation**] Reinforcing healthy qi and eliminating pathogenic factors

Citations

- The therapeutic method of combining yin-fluid nourishment and purging *Chengqi* Decoction (Purgative Decoction) is an important example of reinforcing healthy qi and eliminating pathogenic qi. (*The Simple Treatise on Seasonal Throat Disorders*)
- Supplementing healthy qi should be given top priority in the treatment of a deficiency pattern (deficiency of healthy qi with mild pathogenic qi). Once healthy qi is restored, pathogenic qi can no longer do further harm to the body. Therefore, the therapy involves dispelling pathogenic qi while supplementing healthy qi.... In the treatment of an excess pattern (exuberance of pathogenic qi with no deficiency of healthy qi), expelling pathogenic qi should be prioritized. Once pathogenic qi is removed, health will be automatically restored. (*Comprehensive Medicine by Doctor Zhang Lu*)

90. TIÁOLǏ YĪNYÁNG 调理阴阳

Regulating Yin and Yang

The term refers to adjusting yin-yang disharmony and re-establishing yin-yang balance by reducing the excess and supplementing the deficiency. In traditional Chinese medicine (TCM), yin and yang can be used as an overarching pair for classification or two entity concepts. As classification standards, imbalance between yin and yang covers and explains various pathological changes, including exterior-interior transmission, cold-heat transformation, predominance or debilitation of healthy qi or pathogenic qi, disharmony between nutrient qi and defense qi, and qi-blood imbalance. Therefore, to regulate yin and yang is regarded as the fundamental principle in TCM therapy, including specific sub-principles such as reinforcing healthy qi and eliminating pathogenic qi, regulating the zang-fu organs, regulating qi and blood, harmonizing nutritive and defensive aspects, as well as promoting regular ascending and descending of qi. When yin and yang are regarded as entity concepts, yin-yang imbalance refers to the abnormal state of yin or yang in the human body, that is, predominance, debilitation, mutual impairment, repelling, or even loss of yin or yang, among which predominance or debilitation of yin or yang is the primary etiology. Therefore, in this case, to regulate yin and yang generally refers to the therapeutic principles of reducing the excess or supplementing the deficiency in accordance with the changes in the predominance or debilitation of yin or yang, and combining reducing with supplementing methods, which is usually regarded as the common interpretation of this term.

[**Previous Translation**] Regulation of yin and yang (调整阴阳); coordinate Yin and Yang (调和阴阳)
[**Current Translation**] Regulating yin and yang (调整阴阳); regulating yin and yang; coordinating yin and yang; regulate yin and yang
[**Standard Translation**] Regulating yin and yang

Citations

- This formula tranquilizes the mind and nourishes the spirit. It can regulate yin and yang to restore a balance. (*Orthodoxy of Medicine*)
- Therefore, *Huanglian* Decoction (Coptis Decoction) is used. With a combination of cold and warm, sweet and bitter medicinals in the formula, yin and yang are regulated to achieve harmony. (*Golden Mirror of Medical Tradition*)
- *Shiwei Xiangru* Drink (Ten-ingredient Molsa Drink) works to treat various deficiency patterns resulting from internal damage. It regulates yin and yang, and relieves diarrhea. (*Summary of Key Medical Formula*)

91. YĪNBÌNG ZHÌYÁNG 阴病治阳

Treating Yin Diseases from Yang Aspect

The term means that yang qi should be supplemented to restrict excessive yin in treating deficiency-cold pattern due to relative predominance of yin. It is also known as "warming yang to dissipate cold" or "replenishing the source of fire (yang) to dissipate excessive yin" (*Plain Conversation in Yellow Emperor's Internal Canon of Medicine Annotated by Wang Bing*). Yin and yang restrict each other. When yang is too deficient to restrain yin, yin will become relatively predominant, and various manifestations of deficiency cold may occur. Therefore, in treating the relative predominance of yin, the focus is on the deficient aspect and yang should be supplemented.

[**Previous Translation**] Treat *yang* for *yin* disease; TREATING YANG FOR THE YIN DISEASE; treating yang for yin diseases; treating yin disease from yang aspect; treat Yang for Yin disease

[**Current Translation**] Treating yang for yin disease; treating yang for yin diseases; treating yang to cure yin disease; treating yin disease from yang aspect; yang aspect treated for diseases of the yin nature; yin disease treated through yang

[**Standard Translation**] Treating yin diseases from yang aspect

Citations

• By differentiating whether the disease lies in yin or yang aspect, one can decide what formula should be used. Treat a yin disease from yang aspect, and vice versa. (*Plain Conversation*)
• Relative predominance of yin results from the impairment of yang qi. To treat it, yang qi should be supplemented by warming and tonifying kidney yang. (*Essentials of the Internal Canon of Medicine*)

92. YÁNGBÌNG ZHÌYĪN 阳病治阴

Treating Yang Diseases from Yin Aspect

The term means that yin fluids can be enriched to restrict excessive yang in treating deficiency-heat pattern due to relative predominance of yang. It is also known as "enriching yin fluids to clear heat" or "strengthening the source of water (yin) to restrict hyperactive yang" (*Plain Conversation in Yellow Emperor's Internal Canon of Medicine Annotated by Wang Bing*). Yin and yang restrict each other. When yin is too deficient to restrain yang, yang will become relatively predominant, and various manifestations of deficiency heat may occur. Therefore, in treating relative predominance of yang, the focus is on the deficient aspect and yin should be supplemented.

[**Previous Translation**] Treat *yin* for *yang* disease; treating yin for yang diseases; treating yang disease from yin aspect; treat Yin for Yang disease
[**Current Translation**] Treating yin for the yang disease; treating yin for yang disease; treating yin to cure yang disease; treating yang disease from yin aspect; treating the yin aspect for diseases of yang nature; yang disease treated through yin
[**Standard Translation**] Treating yang diseases from yin aspect

Citations

- Relative predominance of yang results from the damage of yin fluids. To treat it, yin fluids should be supplemented by nourishing the source of yin. (*Essentials of the Internal Canon of Medicine*)
- Yang predominance undoubtedly results in yin deficiency, and vice versa. There are sayings about therapeutic methods as follows: "Treat heat patterns with cold medicinals to purge heat—if heat is unrelieved, treat with yin-nourishing medicinals; treat cold patterns with hot medicinals to dissipate cold—if cold is unrelieved, treat with yang-supplementing medicinals" and "strengthen the source of water to restrict hyperactive yang; replenish the source of fire to dissipate excessive yin." These methods follow the principle of treating yang diseases from yin aspect, and treating yin diseases from yang aspect. (*Original Decrees of Medicine*)

93. YĪN ZHŌNG QIÚ YÁNG 阴中求阳

Obtaining Yang from Yin

The term refers to the addition of yin-enriching medicinals to the yang-tonifying formula in the treatment of yang debilitation. As yin and yang are mutually dependent and rooted, one can make good use of this relationship in composing a formula for the treatment of yang-qi debilitation to achieve better therapeutic effects: mainly use yang-tonifying medicinals and add a few yin-nourishing ones to facilitate the generation and transformation of yang qi. The composition of *You Gui* Pill (Right-Restoring Pill) is a case in point.

[Previous Translation] Treat Yang in Yin
[Current Translation] Obtaining yang from yin; treat yin for yang; treating yin for yang
[Standard Translation] Obtaining yang from yin

Citations

- Doctors adept at the methods of tonifying yang always obtain yang from yin to ensure continuous generation of yang with the addition of yin. Likewise, those good at the methods of nourishing yin obtain yin from yang to ensure abundant generation of yin with the help of yang. (*Jingyue's Complete Works*)
- The rationale for the principles of obtaining yang from yin and obtaining yin from yang is that yin and yang are mutually dependent and rooted. (*Rhymed Discourse on External Remedies*)

94. YÁNG ZHŌNG QIÚ YĪN 阳中求阴

Obtaining Yin from Yang

The term refers to the addition of yang-tonifying medicinals to the yin-enriching formula in the treatment for yin debilitation. As yin and yang are mutually dependent and rooted, one can make good use of this relationship in composing a formula for the treatment of yin-essence debilitation to achieve better therapeutic effects: mainly use yin-nourishing medicinals and add a few yang-tonifying ones to promote the generation and transformation of yin essence. The composition of *Zuo Gui* Pill (Left-Restoring Pill) is a case in point.

[Previous Translation] Getting yin from yang; treat Yin in Yang
[Current Translation] Obtaining yin from yang; treat yang for yin; treating yang for yin
[Standard Translation] Obtaining yin from yang

Citations

- Doctors good at the methods of enriching yin obtain yin from yang to ensure abundant generation of yin with the help of yang. (*Jingyue's Complete Works*)
- Therefore, *Yellow Emperor's Internal Canon of Medicine* says that doctors good at the methods of tonifying yang will obtain yang from yin, while those good at the methods of enriching yin usually obtain yin from yang. (*True Transmission of Medical Principles*)

95. YÌQIÁNG FÚRUÒ 抑强扶弱

Inhibiting the Strong and Supporting the Weak

The term refers to a primary therapeutic principle developed in accordance with the restraining cycle among the five elements. Although abnormal restraining relationships may vary in forms including excess, inadequacy, and counter-restraining, the causes fall into two broad categories—the strong and the weak. When an element is excessively strong, it will manifest signs of hyperfunction. By contrast, hypofunction occurs when one gets excessively weak. Therefore, in treatment, the principle of inhibiting the strong and supporting the weak should be carried out simultaneously, emphasizing either inhibiting the strong to help the weak restore to normal or supporting the weak to avoid being restricted or further aggravation. On the one hand, the principle of inhibiting the strong is applicable to over-restriction or counter-restriction due to excessive restricting. For example, excessive liver (wood) qi over-restricts the spleen and stomach (earth), leading to liver-spleen or liver-stomach disharmony, which is described as excessive wood (liver) over-restricting earth (spleen) and should be treated chiefly by soothing and pacifying liver qi. On the other hand, the principle of supporting the weak is applicable to over-restriction or counter-restriction due to the insufficiency of restriction, such as liver (wood) qi attacking deficient spleen (earth) leading to liver-spleen disharmony, which is described as earth (spleen) deficiency leading to over-restriction by wood (liver) and should be treated chiefly by fortifying spleen qi.

[Previous Translation] /
[Current Translation] Inhibiting the strong and supporting the weak; inhibiting excessiveness (抑强); supporting weakness (扶弱)
[Standard Translation] Inhibiting the strong and supporting the weak

Citations

- Five climatic qi may vary in intensity, and zang-fu organs vary from tenderness to resolution. Therefore, in treatment, the strong should be inhibited and the weak supported so that qi can be regulated to achieve balance. (*Elementary Learning of Medical Canons*)
- Besides, the conditions of *yangming* and *shaoyang* meridians as well as the five zang-organs should be carefully observed regarding predominance and debilitation. By inhibiting the strong and supporting the weak, a harmonious state of qi can be achieved. (*Collected Commentaries on "Treatise on Cold Damage"*)

96. YÌMÙ FÚTǓ 抑木扶土

Inhibiting Wood to Support Earth

The term refers to the therapeutic method of treating liver-spleen disharmony or liver qi attacking the stomach either by soothing the liver and fortifying the spleen or by pacifying liver qi and harmonizing the stomach. It is also known as soothing the liver and fortifying the spleen, or pacifying liver qi and harmonizing the stomach, or regulating the liver and the spleen, or harmonizing the liver and the stomach. According to the correspondence between the five elements and the zang-fu organs, the liver pertains to wood; the spleen and the stomach pertain to earth. Therefore, this term refers to suppressing the hyperactive liver qi to strengthen the deficient spleen-stomach qi. Clinically, this method is used to treat liver-spleen or liver-stomach disharmony due to hyperactive liver (wood) qi over-restricting the spleen and the stomach (earth), or stagnated liver (wood) qi failing to regulate the qi flow of the spleen and the stomach (earth). Representative formulas include *Xiaoyao* Powder (Free Wanderer Powder) and *Tongxie Yaofang* (Important Formula for Painful Diarrhea).

[Previous Translation] /
[Current Translation] /
[Standard Translation] Inhibiting wood to support earth

Citations

- If liver (wood) qi is hyperactive, it will over-restrict spleen (earth) qi.... The rationale behind *Xiao Jianzhong* Decoction (Minor Center-fortifying Decoction) is based on the principle of inhibiting wood to support earth. (*Treatise on Medical Formulas*)
- With the impairment of spleen qi, how can the liver wood not over-restrict the spleen earth? Therefore, the suitable method to promptly address this disorder is inhibiting the wood to support the earth. (*Collected Medical Case Records by Doctor Xu in Four Generations*)

97. ZUǑJĪN PÍNGMÙ 佐金平木

Supporting Metal to Suppress Wood

The term, also known as clearing liver and lung fire, refers to the therapeutic method of suppressing hyperactive liver (wood) qi by directing lung (metal) qi downward. According to the correspondence between the five elements and the zang-fu organs, the lung pertains to metal, and the liver pertains to wood. Supporting metal to suppress wood involves aiding lung qi to descend to relieve the excess of liver qi. Clinically, this method is used to treat hyperactive liver fire affecting the lung's function in purification, manifested as wandering pain in the hypochondrium, panting, a wiry pulse, and so on. Medicinals such as *wuzhuyu* (*Fructus Evodiae*, medicinal evodia fruit), dry-fried *sangbaipi* (*Cortex Mori*, white mulberry root-bark), *sugeng* (*Caulis Perillae*, perilla stem), and *pipaye* (*Folium Eriobotryae*, loquat leaf) are often used to direct lung qi downward to soothe liver qi.

- [Previous Translation] Support the metal (lung) to calm the wood (liver); CALMING THE WOOD BY CLEARING THE METAL; supporting metal to suppress wood; treating the metal to subdue to wood

- [**Current Translation**] Treating the lung (metal) to subdue hyperactivity of the liver (wood); supporting metal to suppress wood; supporting lung to suppress liver; supporting metal to suppress wood
- [**Standard Translation**] Supporting metal to suppress wood

Citations

- The name of *Zuo Jin* Pill (Left Metal Pill) suggests its function, i.e., supporting metal to suppress wood. Specifically, the formula is used to clear liver fire and drain dampness. With certain hot-natured medicinals as the paradoxical assistant in the formula, it works to treat extreme heat pattern. (*Six Essentials of Medicine*)
- To treat the pattern by *Jianzhong* Decoction (Center-fortifying Decoction)... double the dosage of *shaoyao* (*Radix Paeoniae Alba seu Rubra*, white or red peony root) to clear fire and relieve vexation, and use *shengjiang* (*Rhizoma Zingiberis Recens*, fresh ginger) to support metal to suppress wood. (*Collected Writings on the Renewal of "Treatise on Cold Damage"*)
- When *shaoyang* qi is dominant, liver (wood) qi tends to be predominant internally, so *ziyuan* (*Radix et Rhizoma Asteris*, tatarian aster root) should be added to support the lung metal to suppress the liver wood. (*Medical Works from the Shibu House*)

98. XIÈNÁN BǓBĚI 泻南补北

Purging South and Nourishing North

The term refers to the therapeutic method of treating heart-kidney disharmony by reducing heart fire and supplementing kidney water. It is also known as clearing fire and enriching water, or enriching yin and reducing fire, or restoring coordination between the heart and the kidney. According to the correspondence between the five elements and zang-fu organs, and the five elements and directions, the heart corresponds to fire, which pertains to south and the kidney corresponds to water, which pertains to north, hence the term "purging south and nourishing north." Clinically, this method is applicable to heart-kidney (fire-water) disharmony due to insufficient kidney yin and effulgent heart fire. Fire-clearing medicinals, usually bitter, cold, and dry, tend to damage fluids; if used alone, they will result in severer fluid damage. Yin-nourishing medicinals, mostly bitter and cold, if used alone, cannot restrict the fire from flaming upward. Therefore, only by combining fire-clearing and yin-nourishing methods can the effect of restraining fire and generating water be achieved. *Huanglian Ejiao* Decoction (Coptis and Donkey-Hide Gelatin Decoction) stands as a representative formula.

[**Previous Translation**] Purging the south and tonifying the north
[**Current Translation**] Reducing the south while reinforcing the north; purging south and nourishing north; purging heart-fire and nourishing kidney-water
[**Standard Translation**] Purging south and nourishing north

Citations

- The black and dry tongue body indicates fluid exhaustion with internal blazing fire in a patient. The method of purging south and nourishing north should be adopted promptly. (*Treatment of Externally Contracted Warm Febrile Diseases*)
- To enrich yin and reduce fire or to purge south and nourish north is what *zhimu* (*Rhizoma Anemarrhenae*, common anemarrhena rhizome) excels at. (*Treasury of Words on Materia Medica*)
- Promptly enrich the source of yin by purging south (fire) and nourishing north (water) to pacify liver qi so that fetal qi can be tranquilized. (*Profound Scholarship in Gynecology*)

99. PÉITǓ ZHÌSHUǏ 培土制水

Banking Up Earth to Restrain Water

The term refers to the therapeutic method of treating internal accumulation of water and dampness by warming spleen yang or warming the kidney to fortify the spleen. It is also known as the method of regulating earth to remove water, fortifying spleen yang to drain water, or fortifying spleen yang to dispel dampness. According to the correspondence between the five elements and the zang-fu organs, earth refers to the spleen. The word "water" in the term refers to the pathological water or dampness. Clinically, this method is applicable to various disorders manifested as edema, distension, and the feeling of fullness which are due to the overflow of water or dampness as a result of deficient spleen yang failing to transport and transform water normally. Representative formulas include *Shipi Drink*

(Spleen-fortifying Drink) and *Fangji Huangqi* Decoction (Stephania Root and Astragalus Decoction).

[**Previous Translation**] Banking up earth (培土); strengthen Earth to control Water
[**Current Translation**] Tonifying the spleen (earth) to restrain water; banking up earth (培土); banking up earth to control water; supplementing spleen to control bladder
[**Standard Translation**] Banking up earth to restrain water

Citations

* Use *Guizhi* Decoction (Cinnamon Twig Decoction) without g*uizhi* (*Ramulus Cinnamomi*, Cinnamon Twig) but add in *fuling* (*Poria*, poria)… in combination with *gancao* (*Radix et Rhizoma Glycyrrhizae*, licorice root) and *dazao* (*Fructus Jujubae*, Chinese date) to achieve the effect of banking up earth to restrain water. (*Collected Writings on the Renewal of "Treatise on Cold Damage"*)
* In *Fuling Guizhi Gancao Dazao* Decoction (Poria, Cinnamon Twig, Licorice Root, and Chinese Date Decoction)… *guizhi* (*Ramulus Cinnamomi*, Cinnamon Twig) consolidates heart qi, *fuling* (*Poria*, poria) discharges pathogenic kidney qi (water), while *gancao* (*Radix et Rhizoma Glycyrrhizae*, licorice root) and *dazao* (*Fructus Jujubae*, Chinese date) work collaboratively to bank up earth to restrain water. (*Seeking Root Causes of Cold Damage*)
* *Shengjiang* (*Rhizoma Zingiberis Recens*, fresh ginger) diffuses yang qi, while *baizhu* (*Rhizoma Atractylodis Macrocephalae*, white atractylodes rhizome) banks up earth to restrain water. (*Revised Collection of Patterns and Treatments Dated Back to Zhang Zhongjing's "Treatise on Cold Damage"*)

100. BǓMǓ XIÈZǏ 补母泻子

Tonifying Mother Organ and Reducing Child Organ

The term refers to a primary therapeutic principle developed in accordance with the generating cycle among the five elements. According to the mutual-generating principle among the five elements, there exists mother-child relationship among the five zang-organs. The element of "generating" is named as mother organ while that of "being generated" is child organ. Tonifying mother organ suggests that when a zang-organ is in deficiency, apart from supplementing the organ itself, its mother organ could also be strengthened to promote recovery. For example, in the case of liver-blood deficiency, in addition to nourishing the blood of the liver (wood, child organ), the essence of the kidney (water, mother organ) could also be replenished to promote the generation of liver blood. On the other hand, reducing child organ suggests that when a zang-organ is in excess, apart from dispelling the excess pathogenic factors related to the organ itself, its child organ could also be reduced to achieve better effects. For example, with excessive liver fire, in addition to clearing fire of the liver (wood, mother organ), the fire of the heart (fire, child organ) could also be purged to facilitate the elimination of hyperactive liver fire.

[**Previous Translation**] The Combination of Reinforcing Mother Point and Reducing Son Point (补母泻子法)

[**Current   Translation**]   Mother-tonifying   child-reducing   method (补母泻子法)

[**Standard Translation**] Tonifying mother organ and reducing child organ

Citations

- To treat the deficiency pattern of a child organ, one could tonify its mother organ. To treat the excess pattern of a mother organ, one could reduce its child organ. (*Canon of Difficult Issues*)
- The stomach is situated in the middle energizer and distributes body fluids to all other organs. Tonifying the stomach to reduce lung heat therefore follows the rule of tonifying mother organ and reducing child organ. (*Ancient Formulas from the Crimson Snow Garden*)
- The therapeutic method of tonifying mother organ and reducing child organ used by ancient people is perhaps derived from it. For example, if a patient initially has lung-qi deficiency and then is affected by excess pathogenic qi such as wind-heat or phlegm-rheum, one should tonify the spleen and dispel pathogenic qi in the lung instead of simultaneously reinforcing and reducing the lung. (*Random Notes While Reading About Medicine*)

101. PÉITǓ SHĒNGJĪN 培土生金

Banking Up Earth to Generate Metal

The term refers to the therapeutic method of nourishing lung qi by tonifying spleen qi, which is also known as the method of replenishing lung qi by tonifying spleen qi. According to the correspondence between the five elements and the zang-fu organs, the spleen corresponds to earth, and the lung corresponds to metal. Due to the mother-child relationship between them, banking up earth (mother, spleen) can help restore the functions of metal (child, lung). Clinically, this method is used to treat lung-qi deficiency due to the lack of generating source because of spleen-qi deficiency, or to treat qi deficiency of both the lung and the spleen as a result of initial lung-qi deficiency. A representative formula is *Shen Ling Baizhu* Power (Ginseng, Poria, and White Atractylodes Powder).

[**Previous Translation**] Earth up to generate metal (strengthen the spleen to benefit the lung); TONIFYING THE SPLEEN TO HELP THE LUNGS; building up the "earth" to supplement the "metal"; banking up earth to generate metal; strengthen Lung (Metal) by way of reinforcing Spleen (Earth)

[**Current Translation**] Reinforcing the spleen (earth) to strengthen the lung (metal); banking up earth to benefit metal; banking up earth to generate metal; supplementing spleen to strengthen lung; building up earth (spleen) to generate metal (lung)

[**Standard Translation**] Banking up earth to generate metal

Citations

- If the spleen and the stomach are in deficiency, the therapeutic method of banking up earth to generate metal should be used in combination. (*Treatise on Medical Formulas*)
- Some suggest enriching water to clear metal. Others advise banking up earth to generate metal. They all think they treat the root cause of the disease. However, neither method is suitable because the disorder indicates an excess pattern instead of a deficiency one. (*Medical Understanding*)

- Then, use sweet and cool medicinals to bank up earth to generate
  metal. In this way, a strong and healthy state will be restored in one
  month. (*Collection of Case Records in External Patterns*)

102. ZĪSHUǏ HÁNMÙ 滋水涵木

Enriching Water to Moisten Wood

The term refers to the therapeutic method of nourishing liver yin by
enriching kidney yin, which is also known as the method of nourishing the
liver by supplementing the kidney, or enriching and tonifying both the
liver and the kidney. According to the correspondence between the five
elements and the zang-fu organs, the kidney corresponds to water and the
liver corresponds to wood. As water generates wood, there is a mother-
child relationship between the kidney and the liver. When the liver is
affected by kidney-yin deficiency and causes yin deficiency of both the liver
and the kidney, it is described as kidney water failing to moisten liver
wood. To treat it, kidney yin should be supplemented to nourish liver yin
to subdue liver fire and suppress hyperactive liver yang. Clinically, this
method is applicable to the treatment of various liver disorders resulting
from kidney-yin deficiency, for example, liver-yin insufficiency, or even
liver-fire superabundance and liver-yang hyperactivity. Representative formulas include *Da Buyin* Pill (Major Yin-supplementing Pill), *Zhi Bai
Dihuang* Pill (Anemarrhena, Phellodendron, and Rehmannia Pill) and *Qi
Ju Dihuang* Pill (Lycium Berry, Chrysanthemum, and Rehmannia Pill).

[**Previous Translation**] Providing water for the growth of wood; enriching water to nourish wood; replenish Kidney Yin to nourish Liver
[**Current Translation**] Providing water for growth of wood; nourishing
the liver and kidney; enriching water to nourish wood; enrich water to
moisten wood; enrich water to moisten wood; nourishing water to
moisten wood
[**Standard Translation**] Enriching water to moisten wood

Citations

- The therapeutic method of enriching water to moisten wood is used
  to pacify liver yang to extinguish wind. The formula is composed of
  zhigancao (*Radix et Rhizoma Glycyrrhizae Praeparata* cum *Melle*,

prepared licorice root), *dangshen* (*Radix Codonopsis*, codonopsis root), *shudi* (*Radix Rehmanniae Praeparata*, prepared rehmannia root), *maidong* (*Radix Ophiopogonis*, dwarf lilyturf tuber), *ejiao* (*Colla Corii Asini*, donkey-hide gelatin), *zhima* (*Semen Sesami Nigrum*, sesame), *fushen* (*Sclerotium Poriae Pararadicis*, Indian bread with hostwood), *suanzaoren* (*Semen Ziziphi Spinosae*, spiney date seed), *wuweizi* (*Fructus Schisandrae Chinensis*, Chinese magno-livine fruit), *muli* (*Concha Ostreae*, oyster shell), *fuxiaomai* (*Fructus Tritici Levis*, blighted wheat), and *nanzao* (*Fructus Jujubae*, Chinese date). (*Cheng Xingxuan's Case Records*)

• The pattern is stirring of wind due to liver yin deficiency. Therefore, the only available choice is enriching water to moisten wood. There is no other solution. (*Case Records of Ganshan Cottage*)

103. YÌHUǑ BǓTǓ 益火补土

Replenishing Fire to Tonify Earth

The term refers to the therapeutic method of tonifying spleen yang by warming kidney yang, which is also known as fortifying spleen yang by warming kidney yang, warming and supplementing kidney-spleen yang, or replenishing fire to warm earth. According to the correspondence between the five elements and the zang-fu organs, the heart corresponds to fire, and the spleen corresponds to earth. As fire generates earth, there is a mother-child relationship between the heart and the spleen. Therefore, replenishing fire to tonify earth means warming and tonifying heart yang to assist spleen (earth) yang. However, the relationship between heart fire and spleen (earth) yang is rarely mentioned when the theory of *Mingmen* (命门, literally, gate of life) gains popularity. Instead, the method is developed into warming spleen yang by tonifying kidney yang which is applicable to the condition of the spleen failing to transport and transform due to kidney-yang debilitation. Representative formulas include *Sishen* Pill (Four-miracle Pill) and *Zhen Wu* Decoction (True Warrior Decoction).

[Previous Translation] Supplement Fire for tonifying the Earth (Spleen)
[Current Translation] Replenishing fire to generate earth (益火生土);
replenishing fire to nourish earth
[Standard Translation] Replenishing fire to tonify earth

Citations

- Kidney yang and spleen yang are of a mother-child relationship. Kidney yang is what governs the activities of triple energizer and the decomposition of food. Therefore, the composing of any formula to warm and tonify spleen yang follows the principle of supplementing mother organ to reinforce child organ (i.e., replenish fire to tonify earth). (*Essentials of the Internal Canon of Medicine*)
- It is therefore of top priority to regulate authentic qi of the zang-fu organs. By replenishing fire (kidney yang) to tonify earth (spleen yang), yang qi in the middle energizer and the lower energizer will be harmonized. (*Classified Commentaries on Ye Gui's Medical Case Records*)
- *Shayuanjili* Tea (Flattened Milkvetch Seed Tea) … can fortify spleen yang by warming kidney yang and improve appetite by strengthening the stomach. It also improves the health of eyes and ears as well as replenishes essence to improve sexual functions. (*Materia Medica Composed While Living in Mountain*)

104. JĪN SHUǏ XIĀNGSHĒNG 金水相生

Mutual Generation Between Metal and Water

The term refers to the therapeutic method of nourishing yin fluids of the lung and the kidney, which is also known as enriching and nourishing both lung yin and kidney yin. According to the correspondence between the five elements and the zang-fu organs, the lung and the kidney correspond to metal and water respectively, with a mother-child relationship between them. Kidney-lung yin deficiency occurs when lung yin is deficient and fails to nourish kidney yin, or when kidney yin is deficient and fails to nourish lung yin. In this case, both lung yin and kidney yin should be enriched and nourished to promote their mutual generation for better therapeutic effects. Specifically, in the case of metal (lung) failing to generate water (kidney), with signs and symptoms of lung-fluid deficiency first and kidney-yin deficiency later, the main therapeutic method should be supplementing lung yin to nourish kidney yin. Formulae such as *Baihe*

Gujin Decoction (Lily Bulb Metal-securing Decoction) are applicable. If the prominent cause is overconsumption of kidney yin leading to deficient kidney fire flaring up to consume the yin fluids of the lung, the main therapeutic method should be enriching kidney yin. Formulae such as *Mai Wei Dihuang* Pill (Dwarf Lilyturf Tuber, Schisandra and Rehmannia Pill) can be used.

[**Previous Translation**] Generation between metal and water; generation between metal and water; mutual promotion between metal and water

[**Current Translation**] Mutual promotion between lung and kidney; mutual promotion between metal and water; mutual generation between metal (lung) and water (kidney); mutual generation between metal and water

[**Standard Translation**] Mutual generation between metal and water

Citations

- To regulate and cultivate health by addressing the root cause, *Liuwei Dihuang* Pill (Six-ingredient Rehmannia Pill) in combination with *Shengmai* Drink (Pulse-activating Drink) should be taken throughout the year. Besides enriching yin to restrain yang, they work together to bring the miracle of mutual generation of metal and water. (*Commentaries on Ancient and Modern Case Records*)
- For patients with cough, shortness of breath, or even sweating and dry throat in severe cases, the therapeutic method of mutual generation between metal and water should be adopted. (*Treatise on Seasonal Diseases*)
- Thin patients tend to have yin deficiency with hyperactive fire. For treatment, *Liuwei Dihuang* Pill (Six-ingredient Rehmannia Pill) minus *zexie* (*Rhizoma Alismatis*, alisma rhizome) in combination with *Shengmai* Drink (Pulse-activating Drink) should be used to promote mutual generation between metal and water, thus extinguishing fire and relieving phlegm. (*Comprehensive Medicine by Doctor Zhang Lu*)

105. SĀNYĪN ZHÌYÍ 三因制宜

Treating Diseases in Accordance with Three Factors

The term refers to the principle of designing a suitable therapeutic method in accordance with particular seasonal and climatic factors, geographical environment, and the patient's specific condition. Traditional Chinese medicine (TCM) believes that people live in the natural environment and will undoubtedly be affected by various environmental factors. In addition, people may react differently to those influences and present different manifestations as their constitutions vary from person to person. Therefore, the onset, development, and progression of a disease are greatly affected by various factors, especially seasonal and climatic factors, geographical environment, and the patient's specific condition. In clinical practice, apart from analyzing signs and symptoms in detail, doctors should also take into consideration the above-mentioned factors. Only through making a comprehensive analysis of all involved factors can a proper therapeutic method be determined. The concept of treating diseases in accordance with three factors not only embodies the holistic view, but reflects the integration of principle and flexibility in pattern differentiation in TCM.

[**Previous Translation**] Treatment in accordance with three factors (season, locality, and individual); triple pathogenies (三因)

[**Current Translation**] Treatment of disease in accordance with three conditions; three categories of etiological factors (三因); three types of disease causes (三因); three types of etiologic factors (三因); three categories of disease cause (三因)

[**Standard Translation**] Treating diseases in accordance with three factors

Citations

- In the cases of cold damage in the southern area… if it is complicated with summer-heat, *Zhengqi* Powder (Qi-correcting Powder) should be used; if complicated with cold, *Wu Ji* Powder (Five Accumulations Powder) is more suitable. This illustrates the principle of treating diseases in accordance with geographical environment advanced by the doctors of later generations. (*Medical Warnings*)
- In clinical practice, one shall always find a solution if one could design a therapeutic method based on an analysis of the condition, understand its underlying rationale, and determine the treatment in accordance with the season and time. (*Medical Warnings*)

- The therapy may differ due to seasonal changes and differences in individual constitutions, pulse conditions, and other symptoms. Generally, the fundamental principle is to remove stagnation accompanied with tonification to relieve both heat and cough. (*Collective Case Records Conforming Pulse, Pattern, and Formula*)

106. XUÁNHÚ JÌSHÌ 悬壶济世

Hanging Gourd to Help Patients

The term is used to praise life-saving professionals of traditional Chinese medicine. Legend has it that in the Han Dynasty, an epidemic disease attacked the area around Henan province. Many people died, but local doctors had no cure. One day, an old man came and he set up a medicine stand in a lane, hanging a gourd on the door. Stored in the gourd were some medicinal pills that could specifically treat the epidemic disease. With great skill and a kind heart, the old man would offer a pill to anyone who sought help from him and instruct the patient to take it with warm water. Anyone who took his medicine saw immediate effects. Fei Changfang, a native of Runan, observed that the old man would leap into the gourd after people left. Curiously, Fei paid a visit to the old man with prepared dishes and wine and was then taken into the gourd. Since then, Fei was determined to learn skills from the old man, who taught all he knew to him. The two practiced medicine together. Hence, "hanging gourd to help patients" is used by later generations to refer to those who practice medicine.

[**Previous Translation**] /
[**Current Translation**] /
[**Standard Translation**] Hanging gourd to help patients

Citation

- Fei Changfang was a native of Runan. At one time, he was a market administrator. There was an old man in the marketplace selling medicine at a stand with a gourd hanging in front. When the market was closed, he would (transform into smoke and) leap into the gourd. No one in the marketplace was ever able to see this, but Fei could from upstairs. He felt very curious. (*A History of the Later Han Dynasty*)

107. SHÉN SHÈNG GŌNG QIǍO 神圣工巧

Miraculous, Sage, Skilled, and Ingenious

The term describes the four levels of expertise achieved by the doctors of traditional Chinese medicine through four respective diagnostic methods, namely, inspection, listening and smelling, inquiry, and pulse-taking and palpation. According to "The Sixty-First Issue" of *Canon of Difficult Issues*, having the ability to diagnose a disease through inspection is considered miraculous; through listening and smelling, sage; through inquiry, skilled; through pulse-taking and palpation, ingenious. By combining the four diagnostic methods, a doctor can achieve all four levels of expertise.

[Previous Translation] /
[Current Translation] /
[Standard Translation] Miraculous, sage, skilled, and ingenious

Citations

- According to medical classics, diagnosing a disease through inspection is considered miraculous; through listening and smelling, sage; through inquiry, skilled; through pulse-taking, ingenious. (*Canon of Difficult Issues*)
- Without reading *Canon of Difficult Issues* or *Plain Conversation*, how can a doctor understand the four levels of diagnostic expertise (miraculous, sage, skilled, and ingenious), the intricate theory, and the profound rationale? (*Discussion of Pathology Based on Triple Etiology Doctrine*)
- A fool will never understand the four examination methods (inspection, listening and smelling, inquiry, as well as pulse-taking and palpation) or the four corresponding levels of expertise (miraculous, sage, skilled, and ingenious), while a wise person savors them. (*Elementary Learning of Medical Canons*)

108. JŪNCHÉN ZUǑSHǏ 君臣佐使

Monarch, Minister, Assistant, and Guide

The term illustrates metaphorically how a traditional Chinese medicine formula is composed. The "monarch" and the "minister" are officials in ancient China playing different roles in the governance of an empire. They are used to refer to the major medicinal and the assisting drug. A formula is usually composed of monarch, minister, assistant, and guide medicinals. Among them, the monarch medicinal is the major one used to address the main disease or pattern, thus being indispensable in a formula. The minister medicinal is responsible for enhancing the effects of the monarch medicinal, or for addressing the accompanying disease or pattern. The assistant medicinal facilitates the monarch and the minister medicinals for better effects, treats minor symptoms, restrains the toxic or strong properties of the monarch and the minister medicinals, or works as the paradoxical assistant. The guide medicinal directs all medicinals toward the diseased site or harmonizes all medicinals.

[**Previous Translation**] Monarch, minister, assistant, and guide (indicating the different actions of medicines in a prescription); PRINCIPLES, ASSOCIATES, ADJUVENTS, AND MESSENGERS; monarch, minister, assistant, and guide; monarch, minister, adjuvant and dispatcher, key remedy and its adjuvants

[**Current Translation**] Monarch drug in a prescription (君药); ministerial drug (臣药); adjuvant drug (佐药); conductant drug (使药); sovereign [chief], minister [associate], adjuvant [assistant] and courier [guide]; monarch, minister, assistant, and guide; monarch, minister, adjuvant and dispatcher; sovereign, minister, assistant an envoy; principal, subordinate, adjuvant, and guide; chief, deputy, assistant and envoy herbs

[**Standard Translation**] Monarch, minister, assistant, and guide

Citations

- In a formula, the key medicinal addressing the disease is called the monarch medicinal. The one that assists the monarch is the minister medicinal, and the one that coordinates with the minister medicinal is the guide medicinal. (*Plain Conversation*)

- A formula is usually composed of monarch, minister, assistant, and guide medicinals, and can be classified into a large, small, odd, or even one according to the numbers of included medicinals. (*Precious Mirror of Health*)
- In a formula, the medicinals are differentiated as monarch, minister, assistant, and guide. The monarch medicinal, being greatest in quantity, serves the main function in treating the disease. The quantity of the minister medicinal is second to that of the monarch medicinal, and that of the assistant medicinal is even less. The assistant and guide medicinals are determined in accordance with the accompanying signs and symptoms. (*Danxi's Mastery of Medicine*)

109. SÌQÌ WǓWÈI 四气五味

Four Qi and Five Flavors

The term, also known as "qi and flavor" or "nature and flavor," refers to the fundamental theory used to explain the mechanism of traditional Chinese medicinals. With its own qi and flavor, a medicinal is believed to be able to treat specific patterns and will achieve its distinct therapeutic effects. Therefore, a combination of different medicinals can adjust and treat various pathological conditions of the zang-fu organs or organic lesions.

Four qi, also known as the "four natures," refers to the four properties of Chinese medicinals, that is, cold, hot, warm, and cool. It summarizes the properties of medicinals based on their therapeutic effects. Specifically, medicinals for treating heat pattern mostly pertain to cold or cool natures, while those for cold pattern mostly pertain to hot or warm natures. The five flavors refer to sour, bitter, sweet, pungent, and salty tastes. They not only represent the flavors tasted by the tongue, but also reflect the actual functions of the medicinals. According to the theory of traditional Chinese medicine, different flavors of food or medicinals will exert varied effects on the human body. Specifically, the pungent flavor promotes sweating to release the exterior, and moves qi to relieve pain; the bitter flavor clears heat and fire, resolves toxin, purges fire, and dries dampness; the sweet flavor moistens, tonifies, relaxes spasm, and harmonizes the spleen and the stomach; the sour flavor astringes and consolidates; and the salty flavor softens hardness, dissipates masses, and moistens the intestines to promote defecation. Apart from the five flavors, there are also other flavors such as blandness and astringent flavor.

[**Previous Translation**] Four natures of Chinese medicine (cold, hot, warm, and cool) (四气); FOUR PROPERTIES OF DRUGS (四气); FIVE TASTES OF DRUGS (五味); four characters (四气); five tastes (五味); the four natures (四气/性); five kinds of flavor (sour, bitter, sweet, pungent and salty) (五味); four properties of Herbs (四气); four natures of Herbs (四气); five kinds of flavor (sour, bitter, sweet, pungent and salty) (五味); four properties (四气)

[**Current Translation**] Five kinds of tastes (五味); four natures (四气); five tastes (flavors) (五味); four properties and five tastes; four properties and five flavors of herbs; four natures (四气); four nature of drugs (四气); five flavors (五味); four qi (四气); five flavors (五味); four properties (四气)

[**Standard Translation**] Four qi and five flavors

Citations

- Medicinals differ in flavor (sour, salty, sweet, bitter, and pungent) and qi (cold, hot, warm, and cool). They may also differ regarding being toxic or nontoxic. (*Agriculture God's Canon of Materia Medica*)
- The medicinals have five flavors and four qi/natures. For each of the five flavors, it may have the nature of cold, hot, warm or cool. (*Compendium of Materia Medica*)
- How can malpractice occur if one can accurately differentiate the flavor and qi of each medicinal, and compose the formula in accordance with the principle of properly combining monarch, minister, assistant, and guide medicinals? (*Compendium of Materia Medica*)

110. SHĒNGJIÀNG FÚCHÉN 升降浮沉

Ascending, Descending, Floating, and Sinking

The term, as a concept of drug action, is used to describe the direction-related tendencies of pharmacological effects of Chinese medicinals. Generally, *sheng* (升, ascending) indicates the upward movement to lift; *jiang* (降, descending), the downward movement to downbear; *fu* (浮, floating), moving toward the exterior to diffuse; *chen* (沉, sinking), moving toward the interior to store. Ascending, descending, floating, and sinking represent respectively the upward, downward, outward, and inward movement of medicinal effects and are contrary to the tendency of the disease. They can be classified into two pairs, namely, ascending versus descending and floating versus sinking. For each pair, they are different yet overlapping, which makes it difficult to clearly tell them apart. In clinical practice, ascending and floating are often combined, so are descending and sinking. In terms of yin-yang property, ascending and floating pertain to yang, while descending and sinking pertain to yin.

The tendencies of pharmacological effects of Chinese medicinals are inferred according to their effects on the human body. For the medicinals effective in treating diseases in the upper or exterior part or relieving sinking tendency/manifestations, they are labeled as ascending and floating; for those effective in treating diseases in the lower or interior part or directing adverse flow of qi downward, they are labeled as descending and sinking. Generally, ascending and floating medicinals, with the tendency to move upward and outward, work to lift yang, release the exterior, dissipate cold, induce vomiting, open the orifices, and so on; descending and sinking medicinals, with the tendency to move downward and inward, work to subdue hyperactive yang, direct the counterflow of qi downward, purge, promote urination, astringe, and so on.

[**Previous Translation**] Lift, lower, float, sink (referring to action of Chinese materia medica); lifting, lowering, floating, sinking; ascending, descending, floating, sinking; ascending, descending, floating, and sinking

[**Current Translation**] Lifting, lowering, floating, sinking; ascending, descending, floating and sinking; upbearing, downbearing, floating and sinking; ascending and descending, floating and sinking; upbearing, downbearing, floating and sinking

[**Standard Translation**] Ascending, descending, floating, and sinking

Citations

- Ascending, descending, floating, and sinking: a medicinal that is light and hollow tends to float and ascend, while one that is heavy and solid tends to sink and descend. (*Concise Medicinal Principles of Suxian*)

- When prescribing medicines, one should judge whether a medicinal is cold, hot, warm, cool, or neutral, whether its flavor is pungent, sweet, bland, bitter, sour, or salty, whether its moving tendency is ascending, descending, floating, or sinking, and whether it works to diffuse, unblock, tonify, or purge. (*Renzhai's Direct Guidance on Formulas*)
- The sweet flavor fits the golden mean: sweet medicinals can not only ascend, descend, float, and sink, but also harmonize, relieve spasm, tonify, and purge. (*Materia Medica for Decoctions*).

BIBLIOGRAPHY

1. Wong, K. C., & Wu, L.-T. (1936). *History of Chinese Medicine*. National Quarantine Service.
2. Writing Group of *Chinese-English Glossary of Common Terms in Traditional Chinese Medicine* of Guangzhou College of Traditional Chinese Medicine. (1982). *Chinese-English Glossary of Common Terms in Traditional Chinese Medicine* (Han Ying Chang Yong Zhong Yi Ci Hui). Guangdong Science and Technology Press.
3. Shuai, Xuezhong. (1983). *Chinese-English Terminology of Traditional Chinese Medicine* (Han Ying Shuang Jie Chang Yong Zhong Yi Ming Ci Shu Yu). Hunan Science and Technology Press.
4. Ou, Ming. (1986). *Chinese-English Dictionary of Traditional Chinese Medicine* (Han Ying Zhong Yi Ci Dian). Guangdong Science and Technology Press/ Joint Publishing (H.K.).
5. Unschuld, P. U. (1986). *Nan-Jing*. University of California Press.
6. Chinese-English, Chinese-French, Chinese-German, Chinese-Japanese, Chinese-Russian Medical Dictionary Compiling Committee. (1987). *Chinese-English Medical Dictionary* (Han Ying Yi Xue Da Ci Dian). People's Medical Publishing House.
7. Cheng, X. (1987). *Chinese Acupuncture and Moxibustion*. Foreign Languages Press.
8. Bensky, D., & Barolet, R. (1990). *Formulas & Strategies*. Eastland Press.
9. Li, Zhaoguo. (1993). *Introduction to Traditional Chinese Medicine Translation* (Zhong Yi Fan Yi Dao Lun). Northwest University Press.

© The Author(s), under exclusive license to Springer Nature
Singapore Pte Ltd. 2021
L. Zhaoguo et al., *Key Concepts in Traditional Chinese Medicine II*,
https://doi.org/10.1007/978-981-16-2398-1

10.   Liu, Zhanwen. (1994). *Chinese-English Dictionary of Traditional Chinese Medicine* (Han Ying Zhong Yi Yao Xue Ci Dian). Traditional Chinese Medicine Ancient Classics Press.

11.   Wiseman, Nigel. (1995). *English-Chinese Chinese-English Dictionary of Chinese Medicine* (Ying Han Han Ying Zhong Yi Ci Dian). Hunan Science and Technology Press.

12.   Huang, Jialing. (1997). *New Chinese-English Dictionary of Traditional Chinese Medicine* (Zui Xin Han Ying Zhong Yi Ci Dian). Sichuan Lexicographical Press.

13.   Li, Zhaoguo. (1997). *English Translation Skills for Traditional Chinese Medicine* (Zhong Yi Ying Yu Fan Yi Ji Qiao). People's Medical Publishing House.

14.   Shi, Xuemin, & Zhang, Mengchen. (1998). *A Chinese-English Dictionary of Acupuncture and Moxibustion* (Han Ying Shuang Jie Zhen Jiu Da Ci Dian). Huaxia Publishing House.

15.   Zhang, Qiwen, & Sun, Hengshan. (2001). *A Practical Chinese-English Dictionary of Traditional Chinese Medicine* (Shi Yong Han Ying Zhong Yi Ci Dian). Shandong Science and Technology Press.

16.   Wiseman, N., & Ye, F. (2002). *A Practical Dictionary of Chinese Medicine*. People's Medical Publishing House.

17.   Xie, Zhufan. (2002). *Classified Dictionary of Traditional Chinese Medicine* (Xin Bian Han Ying Zhong Yi Yao Fen Lei Ci Dian). Foreign Language Press.

18.   Li, Zhaoguo. (2002). *Concise Chinese-English Dictionary of Traditional Chinese Medicine* (Jian Ming Han Ying Zhong Yi Ci Dian). Shanghai Scientific & Technical Publishers.

19.   Fang, Tingyu, Chen, Feng, & Wang, Mengqiong. (2003). *New Chinese-English Dictionary of Traditional Chinese Medicine* (Xin Han Ying Zhong Yi Xue Ci Dian). China Medical Science Press.

20.   Xie, Zhufan. (2004). *English Translation of Common Terms in Traditional Chinese Medicine* (Zhong Yi Yao Chang Yong Ming Ci Shu Yu Ying Yi). China Press of Traditional Chinese Medicine.

21.   China National Committee for Terms in Science and Technologies. (2004). *Chinese Terms in Traditional Chinese Medicine* (Zhong Yi Yao Xue Ming Ci). Science Press.

22.   World Health Organization Western Pacific Region.   (2007). *WHO International Standard Terminologies on Traditional Medicine in the Western Pacific Region*. Philippines.

23.   World Federation of Chinese Medicine Societies. (2007). *International Standard Chinese-English Basic Nomenclature of Chinese Medicine* (Zhong Yi Ji Ben Ming Ci Shu Yu – Zhong Ying Dui Zhao Guo Ji Biao Zhun). People's Medical Publishing House.

24. Li, Zhaoguo. (2011). *A Concise Chinese-English Dictionary of Yellow Emperor's Canon of Medicine* (Jian Ming Han Ying Huang Di Nei Jing Ci Dian). People's Medical Publishing House.

25. Fang, Tingyu, Ji, Bo, & Wu, Qing. (2013). New Chinese-English Dictionary of Traditional Chinese Medicine, 2nd Ed. (Xin Han Ying Zhong Yi Xue Ci Dian, Di Er Ban). China Medical Science Press. Finally, do I have to click the "Submit" button before July 3 or Zhang Wen of FLTRP will do so? Please let me know it. Thank you for your time.

26. Douglas Wile. (1992). *Art of the Bedchamber: The Chinese Sexual Yoga Classics Including Women's Solo Meditation Texts* (p. 81). New York: State University of New York Press.